The Ultimate Diabetic Recipe Collection

50 wonderful recipes to have fun in the kitchen

Roseann Smith

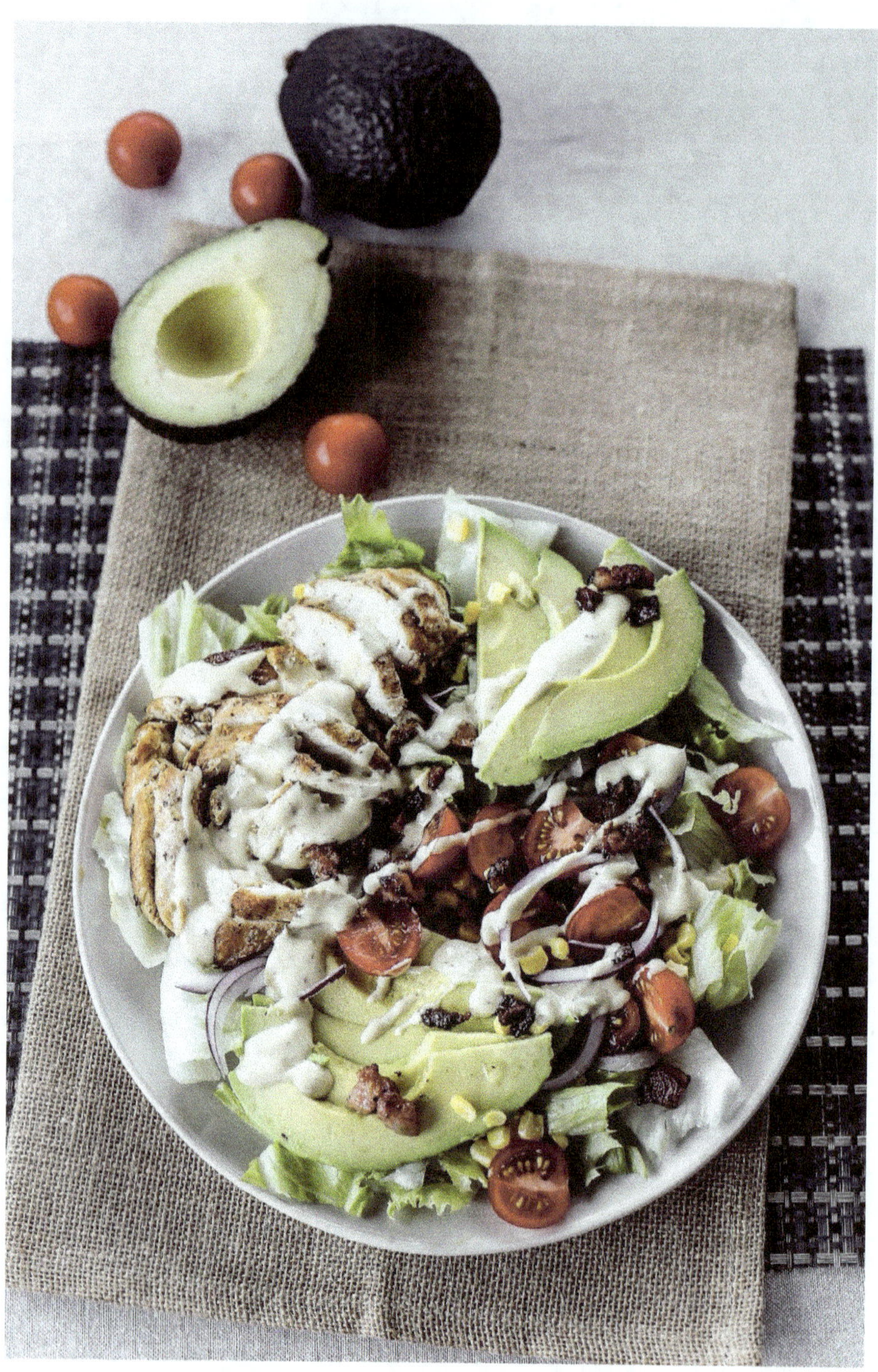

© Copyright 2021 - All rights reserved.

The content contained within this book may not be reproduced, duplicated or transmitted without direct written permission from the author or the publisher.

Under no circumstances will any blame or legal responsibility be held against the publisher, or author, for any damages, reparation, or monetary loss due to the information contained within this book. Either directly or indirectly.

Legal Notice:

This book is copyright protected. This book is only for personal use. You cannot amend, distribute, sell, use, quote or paraphrase any part, or the content within this book, without the consent of the author or publisher.

Disclaimer Notice:

Please note the information contained within this document is for educational and entertainment purposes only. All effort has been executed to present accurate, up to date, and reliable, complete information. No warranties of any kind are declared or implied. Readers acknowledge that the author is not engaging in the rendering of legal, financial, medical or professional advice. The content within this book has been derived from various sources. Please consult a licensed professional before attempting any techniques outlined in this book.

By reading this document, the reader agrees that under no circumstances is the author responsible for any losses, direct or indirect, which are incurred as a result of the use of information contained within this document, including, but not limited to, — errors, omissions, or inaccuracies.

Table of Contents

1. Garden Salad Wraps 6

2. Roasted Eggplant Spread 9

3. Chocolate Muffins... 11

4. Dark Chocolate Cake 15

5. Strawberry & Watermelon Pops 17

6. Raspberry Almond Tart 19

7. Oatmeal Butterscotch Cookies 22

8. Avocado Mousse 24

9. Flourless Chocolate Cake 26

10.   Berry Almond Parfait 29

11.   Homemade Ice Cream Cake 31

12.   Cappuccino Cupcakes 33

13.   Quail Eggs & Prosciutto Wraps 35

14.   Pumpkin Spiced Almonds..................................... 36

15.   Pumpkin Custard.. 37

16.   Peppers And Hummus 39

17.   Strawberry Shake.. 41

18.   Cinnamon Protein Bars 42

19.   Chocó Cookies.. 43

20.   Chocolate Avocado Ice Cream 46

21.   Marinated Strawberries 48

22.   Tomato & Cheese In Lettuce Packets.................... 50

23.   Tofu & Chia Seed Pudding.................................... 51

24.   Mango Mousse 53

25.   Nutty Wild Rice Salad 55

26.	Banana Split Sundae	57
27.	Tzatziki Dip With Cauliflower	59
28.	Plum & Pistachio Snack	61
29.	Fruity Tofu Smoothie	62
30.	Strawberry Mousse	63
31.	Raisin Apple Cake	65
32.	Avocado And Tempeh Bacon Wraps	67
33.	Coco-macadamia Fat Bombs	69
34.	Chocolate-covered Prosecco Strawberries	71
35.	Pumpkin Spice Snack Balls	74
36.	Chocolatey Banana Shake	76
37.	Chia Strawberry Pudding	77
38.	Chocolate Banana Cake	79
39.	Delicious Egg Cups With Cheese & Spinach	82
40.	Lemon Custard	84
41.	Yogurt Cheesecake	86
42.	Fruit Salad	89
43.	Risotto Bites	91
44.	Grilled Avocado Hummus Paninis	94
45.	Cauliflower Muffin	96
46.	Bok Choy Soup	98
47.	Stuffed Mushrooms	100
48.	Roasted Salmon With Lemon	102
49.	White Spinach Pizza With Cauliflower Crust	104
50.	Chickpea, Tuna, And Kale Salad	106

Garden Salad Wraps

Servings: 4

Cooking Time: 10 Minutes

Ingredients:

- 6 tablespoons extra-virgin olive oil
- 1-pound extra-firm tofu, drained, patted dry, and cut into ½-inch strips
- 1 tablespoon soy sauce
- ¼ cup apple cider vinegar
- 1 teaspoon yellow or spicy brown mustard
- ½ teaspoon salt
- ¼ teaspoon freshly ground black pepper
- 3 cups shredded romaine lettuce
- 3 ripe Roma tomatoes, finely chopped
- 1 large carrot, shredded
- 1 medium English cucumber, peeled and chopped
- ⅓ cup minced red onion

- ¼ cup sliced pitted green olives
- 4 (10-inch) whole-grain flour tortillas or lavish flatbread

Directions:

1. Preparing the Ingredients
2. Cook the tofu until golden brown in a large skillet with Over medium heat. Sprinkle with soy sauce and set aside to cool.
3. In a small bowl, combine the vinegar, mustard, salt and pepper with the remaining 4 tablespoons oil, stirring to blend well. Set aside.
4. Finish and Serve
5. combine the cucumber, onion, lettuce, tomatoes, carrot, and olives in a large bowl. Pour on the dressing.
6. Put 1 tortilla on a work surface and spread with about one-quarter of the salad. Place a few strips of tofu on the tortilla and roll up tightly. Slice in half.

Nutrition Info: 191 Cal 16.6 g Fats 9.6 g Protein 0.8 g Net Carb 0.2 g Fiber

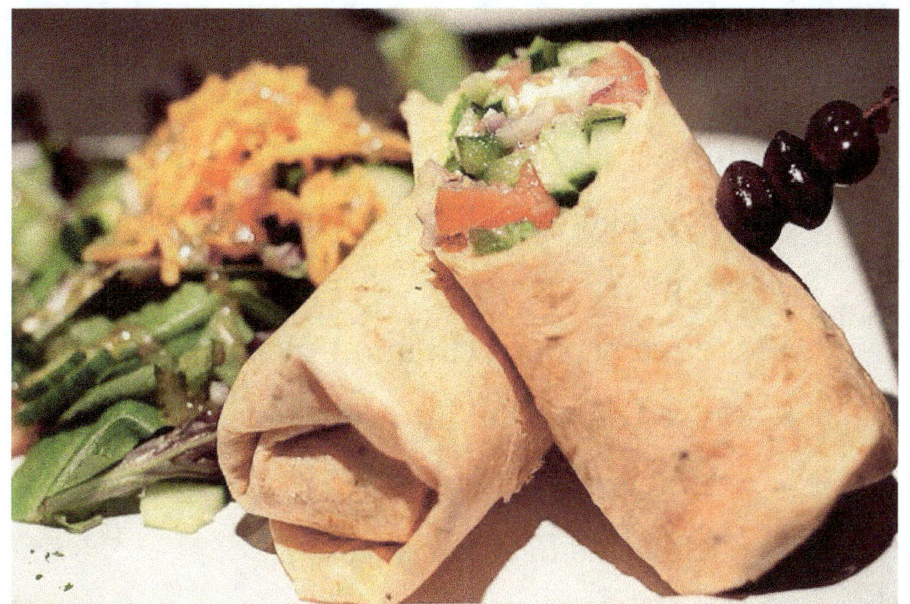

Roasted Eggplant Spread

Servings: 2

Cooking Time: 20 Minutes

Ingredients:

- 1 eggplant, medium, cut into small 1 inch pieces
- 2 red peppers, cut into 1-inch pieces
- 1 red onion, cut into 1-inch pieces
- 1 tablespoon tomato
- 4 toasted baguette slices
- What you will need from the store cupboard:
- 3 garlic cloves, minced
- 3 tablespoons of olive oil
- ½ teaspoon pepper
- ½ teaspoon salt
- Cooking spray

Directions:

1. Preheat your oven to 350 ºF.
2. Mix the olive oil, cloves, salt, and pepper.
3. Keep vegetables in your bowl. Now toss with the oil mix.
4. Transfer to your baking pan where you have applied cooking spray
5. Roast the vegetables till they get soft and are slightly brown.
6. Now keep in a food processor.
7. Add the tomato and pulse until it blends. The mixture must be chunky.
8. Transfer to your bowl. Serve with the baguette.

Nutrition Info: Calories 84 Carbohydrates 9g Fiber 3g Sugar 0.5g Cholesterol 0mg Total Fat 5g Protein 1g

Chocolate Muffins

Servings: 8

Cooking Time: 30 Minutes

Ingredients:

- Pumpkin, chopped, steamed: 2 cups
- Coconut flour: 1/2 cup
- Salt: 1/8 teaspoon
- Erythritol sweetener: 4 tablespoons
- Cacao powder, unsweetened: 1 cup
- Collagen protein powder: 1/2 cup
- Baking soda: 1 teaspoon
- Cacao butter, melted: 4.6 ounces
- Avocado oil: 1/2 cup
- Apple cider vinegar: 2 teaspoons
- Vanilla extract, unsweetened: 3 teaspoons
- Eggs, pastured: 3

Directions:

1. Set oven to 350 degrees F and let preheat until muffins are ready to bake.

2. Add all the ingredients in a food processor or blender, except for collagen, and pulse for 1 to 2 minutes or until well combined and incorporated.

3. Then add collagen and pulse at low speed until just mixed.

4. Take an eight cups silicon muffin tray, grease the cups with avocado oil and then evenly scoop the batter in them.

5. Place the muffin tray into the oven and bake the muffins for 30 minutes or until thoroughly cooked and a knife inserted into each muffin comes out clean.

6. When done, let muffins cool in the pan for 10 minutes, then take them out from the tray and cool on the wire rack.

7. Place muffins in a large freezer bag or wrap each muffin with a foil and store them in the

refrigerator for four days or in the freezer for
up to 3 months.

8. When ready to serve, microwave muffins for
45 seconds to 1 minute or until thoroughly
heated and then serve with coconut cream.

Nutrition Info: Calories: 111 Fat: 9.9 g Protein: 2.8 g
Net Carbs: 3 g Fiber: 1 g

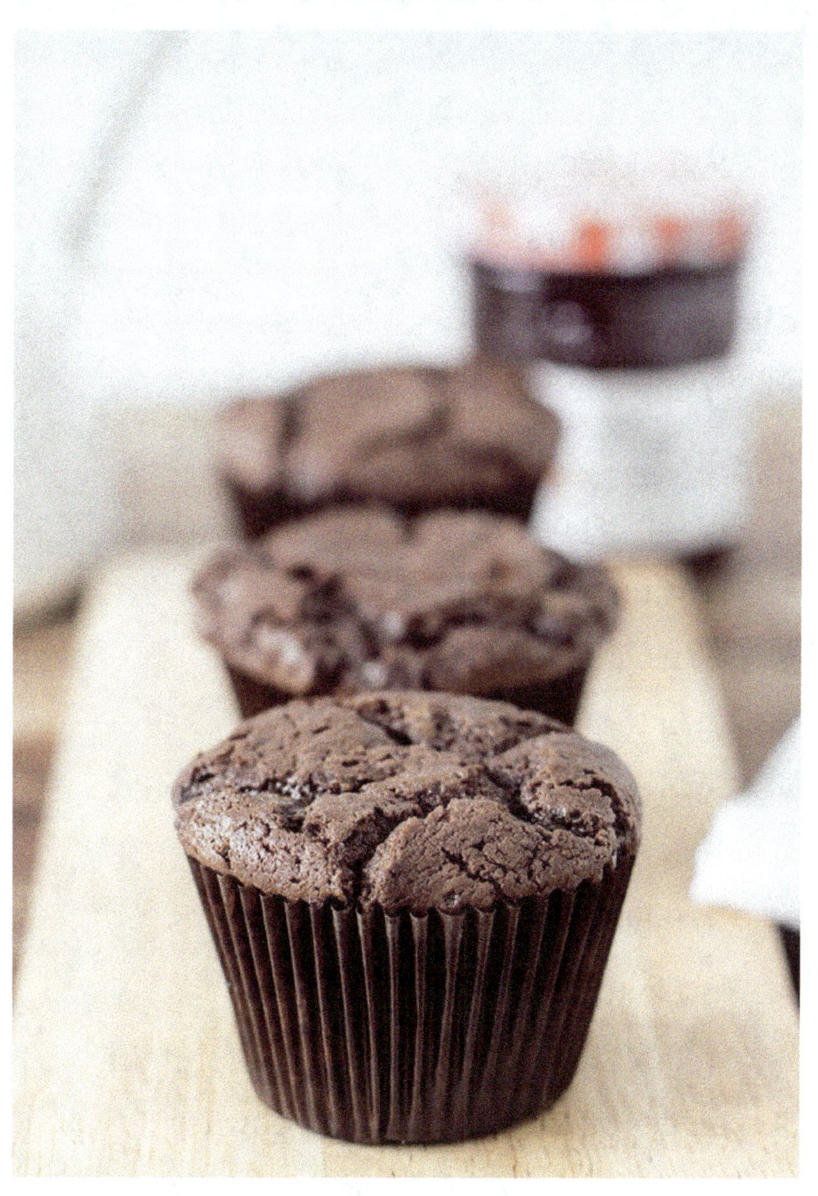

Dark Chocolate Cake

Servings: 10

Cooking Time: 3 Hours

Ingredients:

- 1 cup almond flour
- 3 eggs
- 2 tablespoons almond flour
- 1/4 teaspoon salt
- 1/2 cup Swerve Granular
- 3/4 teaspoon vanilla extract
- 2/3 cup almond milk, unsweetened
- 1/2 cup cocoa powder
- 6 tablespoons butter, melted
- 1 1/2 teaspoon baking powder
- 3 tablespoon unflavored whey protein powder or egg white protein powder
- 1/3 cup sugar-free chocolate chips, optional

Directions:

1. Grease the slow cooker well.

2. Whisk the almond flour together with cocoa powder, sweetener, whey protein powder, salt and baking powder in a bowl. Then stir in butter along with almond milk, eggs and the vanilla extract until well combined, and then stir in the chocolate chips if desired.

3. When done, pour into the slow cooker. Allow to cook for 2-2 1/2 hours on low.

4. When through, turn off the slow cooker and let the cake cool for about 20-30 minutes.

5. When cooled, cut the cake into pieces and serve warm with lightly sweetened whipped cream. Enjoy!

Nutrition Info: 205 calories; 17 g fat; 8.4 g total carbs; 12 g protein

Strawberry & Watermelon Pops

Servings: 6

Cooking Time: 0 Minutes

Ingredients:

- ¾ cup strawberries, sliced
- 2 cups watermelon, cubed
- ¼ cup lime juice
- 2 tablespoons brown sugar
- ⅛ teaspoon salt

Directions:

1. Put the strawberries inside popsicle molds.
2. In a blender, pulse the rest of the ingredients until well mixed.
3. Pour the puree into a sieve before pouring into the molds.
4. Freeze for 6 hours.

Nutrition Info: Calories 57 Total Fat 0 g Saturated Fat 0 g Cholesterol 0 mg Sodium 180 mg Total

Carbohydrate 14 g Dietary Fiber 2 g Total Sugars 11 g
Protein 1 g Potassium 180 mg

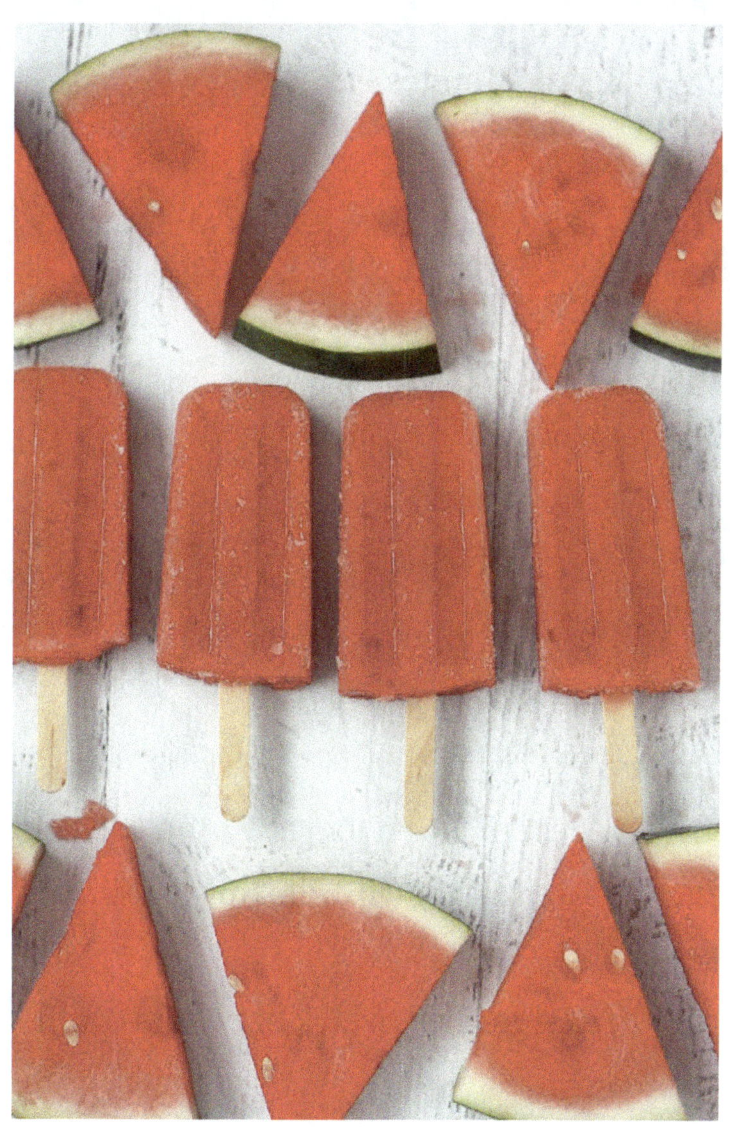

Raspberry Almond Tart

Servings: 4

Cooking Time: 23 Minutes

Ingredients:

- 5 egg whites
- 1 tsp vanilla
- 1 1/2 cups raspberries
- 1 lemon zest, grated
- 1 cup almond flour
- 1/2 cup Swerve
- 1/2 cup butter, melted
- 1 tsp baking powder

Directions:

1. Preheat the oven to 375 F/ 190 C.
2. Grease tart tin with cooking spray and set aside.
3. In a large bowl, whisk egg whites until foamy.

4. Add sweetener, baking powder, vanilla, lemon zest, and almond flour and mix until well combined.

5. Add melted butter and stir well.

6. Pour batter in tart tin and top with raspberries.

7. Bake in preheated oven for 20-23 minutes.

8. Serve and enjoy.

Nutrition Info: Calories 378 Fat 8 g Carbohydrates 14 g Sugar 4 g Protein 11 g Cholesterol 0 mg

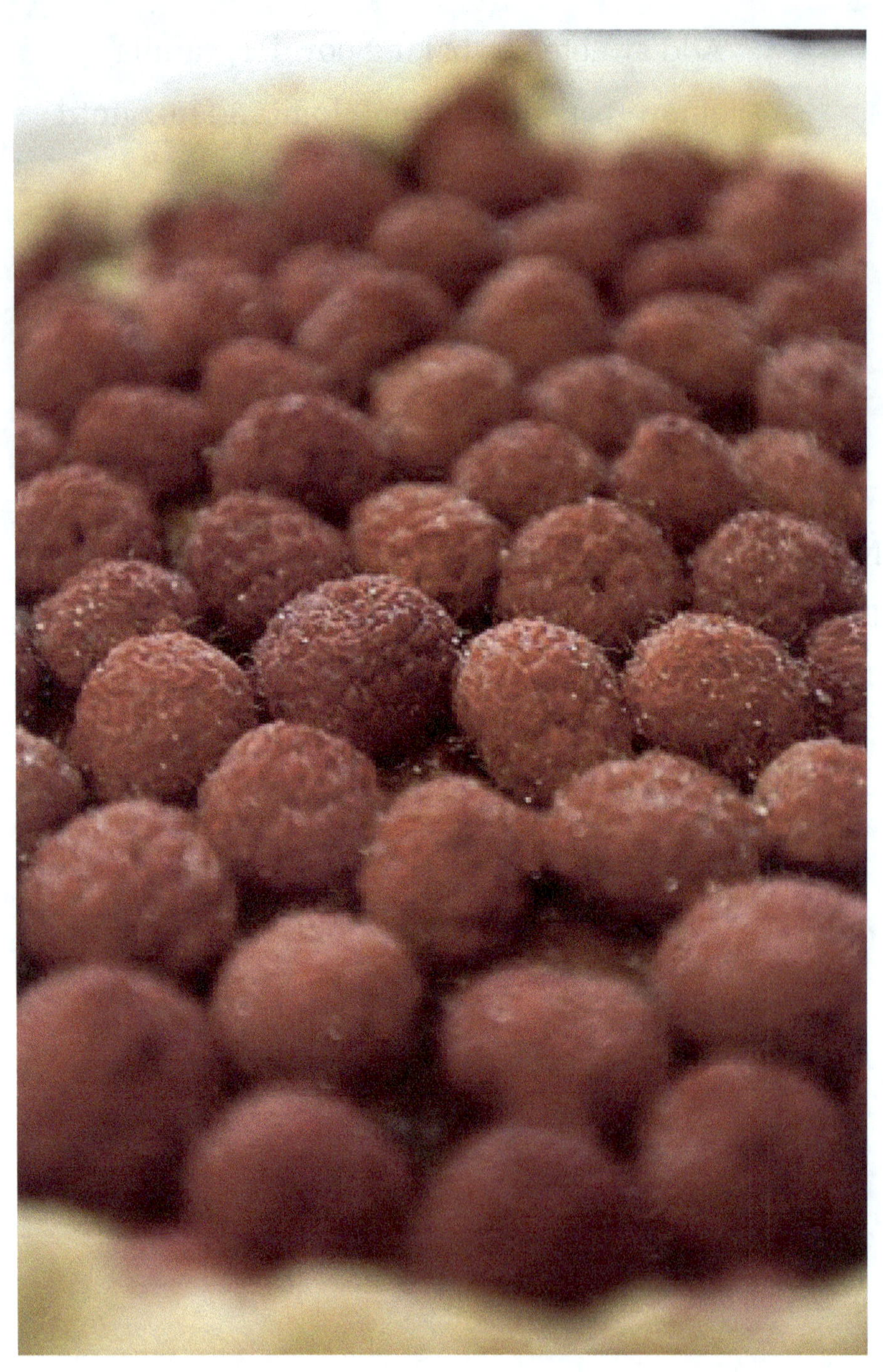

Oatmeal Butterscotch Cookies

Servings: 4 Dozen

Cooking Time: 15 Minutes

Ingredients:

- ½ teaspoon cinnamon, ground
- 3 cups oats
- 2 eggs
- What you will need from the store cupboard:
- 1 teaspoon of baking soda
- 1-1/4 all-purpose flour
- 1 cup margarine or butter
- 1 teaspoon vanilla extract
- ½ teaspoon salt

Directions:

1. Preheat your oven to 350 °F.
2. Bring together the baking soda, flour, salt and cinnamon in a bowl.

3. Beat the eggs, vanilla extract and butter in a mixer bowl.

4. Beat in the flour mix gradually.

5. Stir in the oats.

6. Place rounded tablespoons on baking sheets. Bake for 5-6 minutes.

7. Let it cool for a couple of minutes.

Nutrition Info: Calories 130 Carbohydrates 16g Cholesterol 20mg Fat 7g Protein 1g Sodium 90mg

Avocado Mousse

Servings: 3

Ingredients:

- 2 ripe Haas avocados, peeled, pitted and chopped roughly
- 1 teaspoon liquid stevia
- 1 teaspoon organic vanilla extract
- Pinch of salt

Directions:

1. In a high-speed blender, add all the ingredients and pulse until smooth.
2. Transfer the pudding into a serving bowl.
3. Cover the bowl and refrigerate to chill for at least 2 hours before serving.
4. Meal Prep Tip: Transfer the mousse into an airtight container. Cover the containers and refrigerate for about 1 day.

Nutrition Info: Calories 277 Total Fat 26.1 g Saturated Fat 5.5 g Cholesterol 0 mg Total Carbs 11.7 g Sugar 0.9 g Fiber 8 g Sodium 59 mg Potassium 652 mg Protein 2.6g

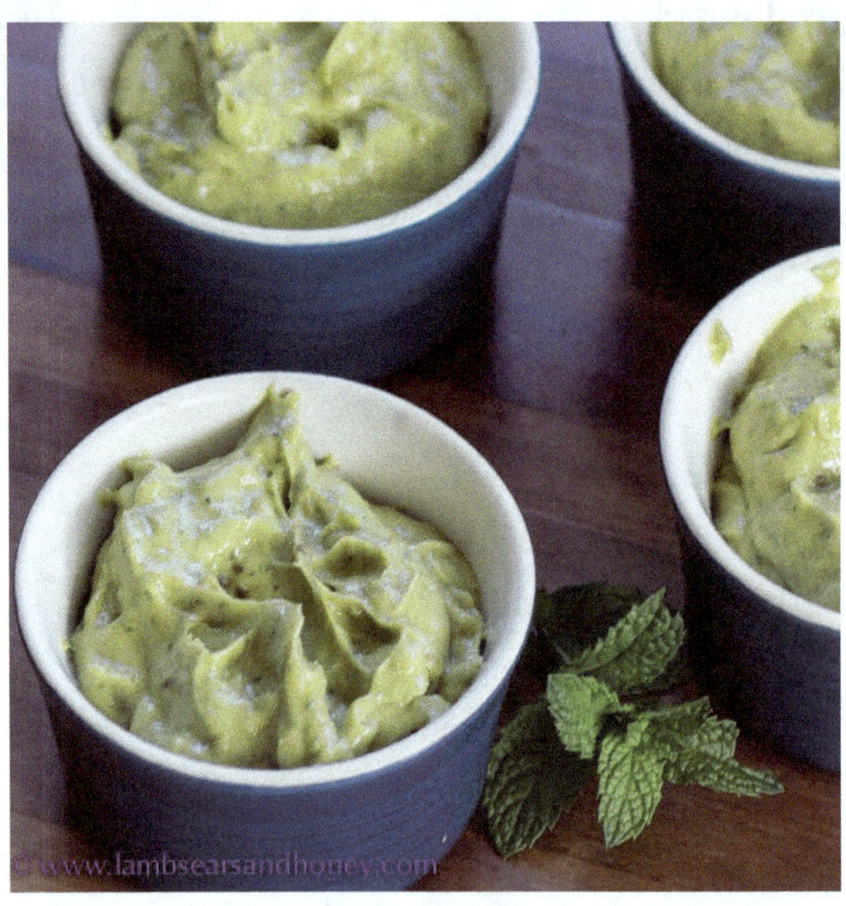

Flourless Chocolate Cake

Servings: 6

Cooking Time: 45 Minutes

Ingredients:

- 1/2 Cup of stevia
- 12 Ounces of unsweetened baking chocolate
- 2/3 Cup of ghee
- 1/3 Cup of warm water
- ¼ Teaspoon of salt
- 4 Large pastured eggs
- 2 Cups of boiling water

Directions:

1. Line the bottom of a 9-inch pan of a spring form with a parchment paper.

2. Heat the water in a small pot; then add the salt and the stevia over the water until wait until the mixture becomes completely dissolved.

3.   Melt the baking chocolate into a double boiler or simply microwave it for about 30 seconds.

4.   Mix the melted chocolate and the butter in a large bowl with an electric mixer.

5.   Beat in your hot mixture; then crack in the egg and whisk after adding each of the eggs.

6.   Pour the obtained mixture into your prepared spring form tray.

7.   Wrap the spring form tray with a foil paper.

8.   Place the spring form tray in a large cake tray and add boiling water right to the outside; make sure the depth doesn't exceed 1 inch.

9.   Bake the cake into the water bath for about 45 minutes at a temperature of about 350 F.

10.   Remove the tray from the boiling water and transfer to a wire to cool.

11. Let the cake chill for an overnight in the refrigerator.

12. Serve and enjoy your delicious cake!

Nutrition Info: Calories: 295| Fat: 26g | Carbohydrates: 6g | Fiber: 4g |Protein: 8g

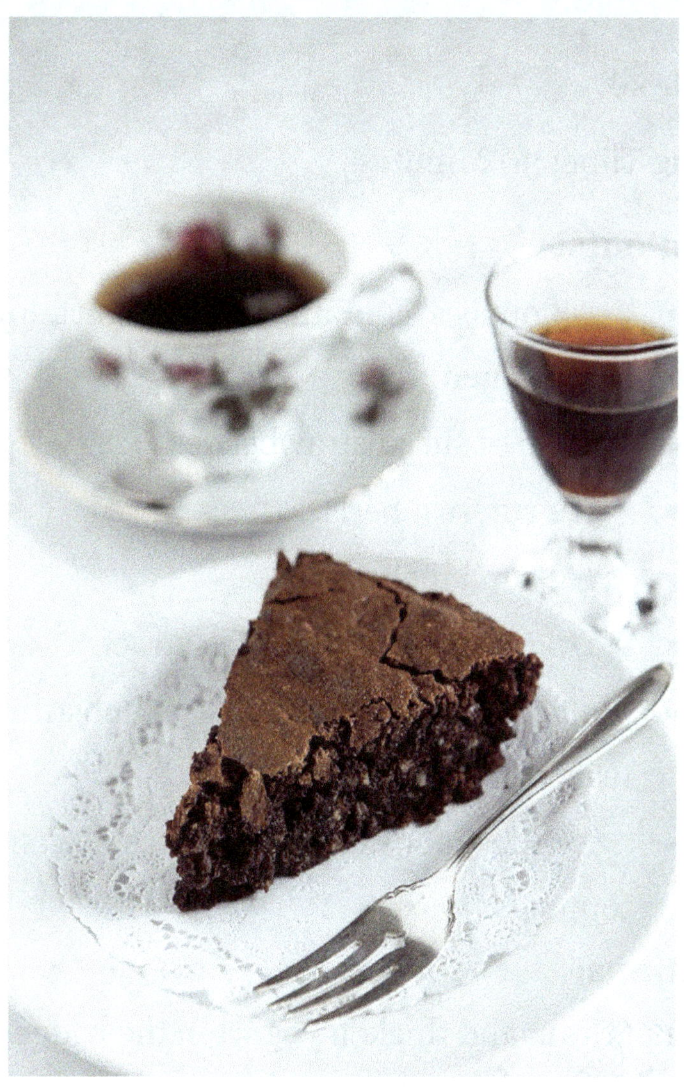

Berry Almond Parfait

Servings: 4

Cooking Time: 30 Minutes

Ingredients:

- 1-8 ounces' container plain yogurt, low-fat and drained
- 1 cup of sliced strawberries
- 1/2 cup raspberries
- 1/2 cup blueberries
- 1/8 teaspoon of almond extract
- 1 tablespoon pourable sugar substitute + 2 teaspoons, divided
- 2 tablespoons toasted slivered almonds for toppings

Directions:

1. Drain and thicken yogurt in the fridge using a paper towel lined strainer for 2 hours to 24 hours. (Do this the night before).

2. Combine all ingredients but using only 2-teaspoon sugar substitute. Toss lightly to mix. Chill for 30 minutes to 2 hours.

3. Transfer the drained yogurt to a bowl and stir in the remaining sugar substitute.

4. Layer 1/3 cup of berries mixture and half yogurt alternately in 2 parfait glasses.

5. Top with almonds to serve.

Nutrition Info: Calories: 220 Carbohydrates: 30 g Fiber: 6 g Fats: 6 g Sodium: 84 mg Protein: 9 g

Homemade Ice Cream Cake

Servings: 4

Cooking Time: 15 Minutes

Ingredients:

- 5 sugar cones, crushed
- 3 tablespoons melted unsalted butter
- 4 cups light ice cream, no-sugar-added and softened, divided
- 1-8 ounces' container whipped topping, reduced-fat and frozen thawed

Directions:

1. Grease a deep pie pan dish with cooking spray.
2. Crush sugar cones in a sealed bag using a rolling pin. Place in a bowl. Stir in the butter until evenly moistened. Use the mixture as your crust. Press onto the bottom of the pan and refrigerate for 20 minutes.

3. Layer 2 cups of the light ice cream over the crust and freeze for 30 minutes or until firm.

4. Spread the remaining light ice cream on top of the frozen first layer and freeze again for another 30 minutes.

5. Spread the whip topping on top then freeze for 2 hours or until it is firm.

6. Let ice cream cake soften for 15 to 30 minutes inside the fridge before slicing and serving.

Nutrition Info: Calories: 118 Carbohydrates: 15 g Fiber: 1 g Fats: 5 g Sodium: 35 mg Protein: 2 g

Cappuccino Cupcakes

Servings: 17

Cooking Time: 15 Minutes

Ingredients:

- 2 eggs
- 2 cups all-purpose flour
- ¼ cup instant coffee granules
- ½ cup of baby food
- ½ cup cocoa, crushed
- What you will need from the store cupboard:
- ¼ cup canola oil
- 1 teaspoon of baking soda
- 2 teaspoons vanilla extract
- ½ teaspoon salt
- 1-1/2 cups low-fat whipped topping
- ½ cup hot water

Directions:

1. Bring together the cocoa, flour, salt, and baking soda in your bowl.
2. Dissolve the coffee granules in hot water.
3. Now whisk together the baby food, eggs, coffee mix, and vanilla in a bowl.
4. Stir the dry ingredients in gradually.
5. Fill into your muffin cups.
6. Bake for 10 to 12 minutes.
7. Sprinkle with cocoa and add the whipped toppings before serving.

Nutrition Info: Calories 192, Carbohydrates 33g, Fiber 1g, Sugar 2g, Cholesterol 22mg, Total Fat 5g, Protein 3g

Quail Eggs & Prosciutto Wraps

Servings: 2

Cooking Time: 10 Minutes

Ingredients:

- 3 thin prosciutto slices
- 9 basil leaves
- 9 quail eggs

Directions:

1. Cover the quail eggs with salted water and bring to a boil over medium heat for 2-3 minutes. Place the eggs in an ice bath and let cool for 10 minutes, then peel them.
2. Cut the prosciutto slices into three strips. Place basil leaves at the end of each strip. Top with a quail egg. Wrap in prosciutto, secure with toothpicks and serve.

Nutrition Info: Calories 243 Fat: 21g Net Carbs: 0.5g Protein: 12.5g

Pumpkin Spiced Almonds

Servings: 4

Cooking Time: 25 Minutes

Ingredients:

- 1 tablespoon olive oil
- 1 ¼ teaspoon pumpkin pie spice
- Pinch salt
- 1 cup whole almonds, raw

Directions:

1. Preheat the oven to 300°F and line a baking sheet with parchment.
2. Whisk together the olive oil, pumpkin pie spice, and salt in a mixing bowl.
3. Toss in the almonds until evenly coated, then spread on the baking sheet.
4. Bake for 25 minutes then cool completely and store in an airtight container.

Nutrition Info: 170 calories 15.5g fat 5g protein 5.5g carbs 3g fiber 2.5g net carbs

Pumpkin Custard

Servings: 6

Cooking Time: 2 Hours 30 Minutes

Ingredients:

- 1/2 cup almond flour
- 4 eggs
- 1 cup pumpkin puree
- 1/2 cup stevia/erythritol blend, granulated
- 1/8 teaspoon sea salt
- 1 teaspoon vanilla extract or maple flavoring
- 4 tablespoons butter, ghee, or coconut oil melted
- 1 teaspoon pumpkin pie spice

Directions:

1. Grease or spray a slow cooker with butter or coconut oil spray.
2. In a medium mixing bowl, beat the eggs until smooth. Then add in the sweetener.

3. To the egg mixture, add in the pumpkin puree along with vanilla or maple extract.

4. Then add almond flour to the mixture along with the pumpkin pie spice and salt. Add melted butter, coconut oil or ghee.

5. Transfer the mixture into a slow cooker. Close the lid. Cook for 2-2 ¾ hours on low.

6. When through, serve with whipped cream, and then sprinkle with little nutmeg if need be. Enjoy!

7. Set slow-cooker to the low setting. Cook for 2-2.45 hours, and begin checking at the two hour mark. Serve warm with stevia sweetened whipped cream and a sprinkle of nutmeg.

Nutrition Info: 147 calories; 12 g fat; 4 g total carbs; 5 g protein

Peppers And Hummus

Servings: 4

Cooking Time: 0 Minutes

Ingredients:

- one 15-ounce can chickpeas, drained and rinsed
- juice of 1 lemon, or 1 tablespoon lemon juice
- ¼ cup tahini
- 3 tablespoons extra-virgin olive oil
- ½ teaspoon ground cumin
- 1 tablespoon water
- ¼ teaspoon paprika
- 1 red bell pepper, sliced
- 1 green bell pepper, sliced
- 1 orange bell pepper, sliced

Directions:

1. Preparing the Ingredients
2. In a food processor, combine chickpeas, lemon juice, tahini, 2 tablespoons of the olive oil, the cumin, and water.
3. Finish and Serve
4. Process on high speed until blended for about 30 seconds. Scoop the hummus into a bowl and drizzle with the remaining tablespoon of olive oil. Sprinkle with paprika and serve with sliced bell peppers.

Nutrition Info: Fat: 10 g Protein: 5.4 g Carbohydrates: 22.8 g

Strawberry Shake

Servings: 2

Cooking Time: 10 Minutes

Ingredients:

- 1½ cups fresh strawberries, hulled
- 1 large frozen banana, peeled
- 2 scoops unsweetened vegan vanilla protein powder
- 2 tablespoons hemp seeds
- 2 cups unsweetened hemp milk

Directions:

1. In a high-speed blender, place all the ingredients and pulse until creamy.
2. Pour into two glasses and serve immediately.

Nutrition Info: Calories 325 Total Fat 13 g Saturated Fat 0.8 g Cholesterol 0 mg Sodium 391 mg Total Carbs 23.3 g Fiber 3.9 g Sugar 12.5 g Protein 31.2 g

Cinnamon Protein Bars

Servings: 8

Cooking Time: 10 Minutes

Ingredients:

- 2 scoops vanilla protein powder
- 1/4 cup coconut oil, melted
- 1 cup almond butter
- 1/4 tsp cinnamon
- 12 drops liquid stevia
- Pinch of salt

Directions:

1. In a bowl, mix together all ingredients until well combined.
2. Transfer bar mixture into a baking dish and press down evenly.
3. Place in refrigerator until firm.
4. Slice and serve.

Nutrition Info: Calories 99 Fat 8 g Carbohydrates 0.6 g Sugar 0.2 g Protein 7.2 g Cholesterol 0 mg

Chocó Cookies

Servings: 14

Cooking Time: 10 Minutes

Ingredients:

- 1 egg
- 1/2 cup erythritol
- 1/4 cup unsweetened cocoa powder
- 1 cup almond butter
- 3 tbsp unsweetened almond milk
- 1/4 cup unsweetened chocolate chips

Directions:

1. Preheat the oven to 350 F/ 180 C.
2. Line baking tray with parchment paper and set aside.
3. In a bowl, mix together almond butter, egg, sweetener, almond milk, and cocoa powder until well combined.
4. Stir in Chocó chips.

5. Make cookies from mixture and place on a
    baking tray.

6. Bake for 10 minutes.

7. Allow to cool completely then serve.

Nutrition Info: Calories 44 Fat 3.5 g Carbohydrates
2.2 g Sugar 0.1 g Protein 1.5 g Cholesterol 12 mg

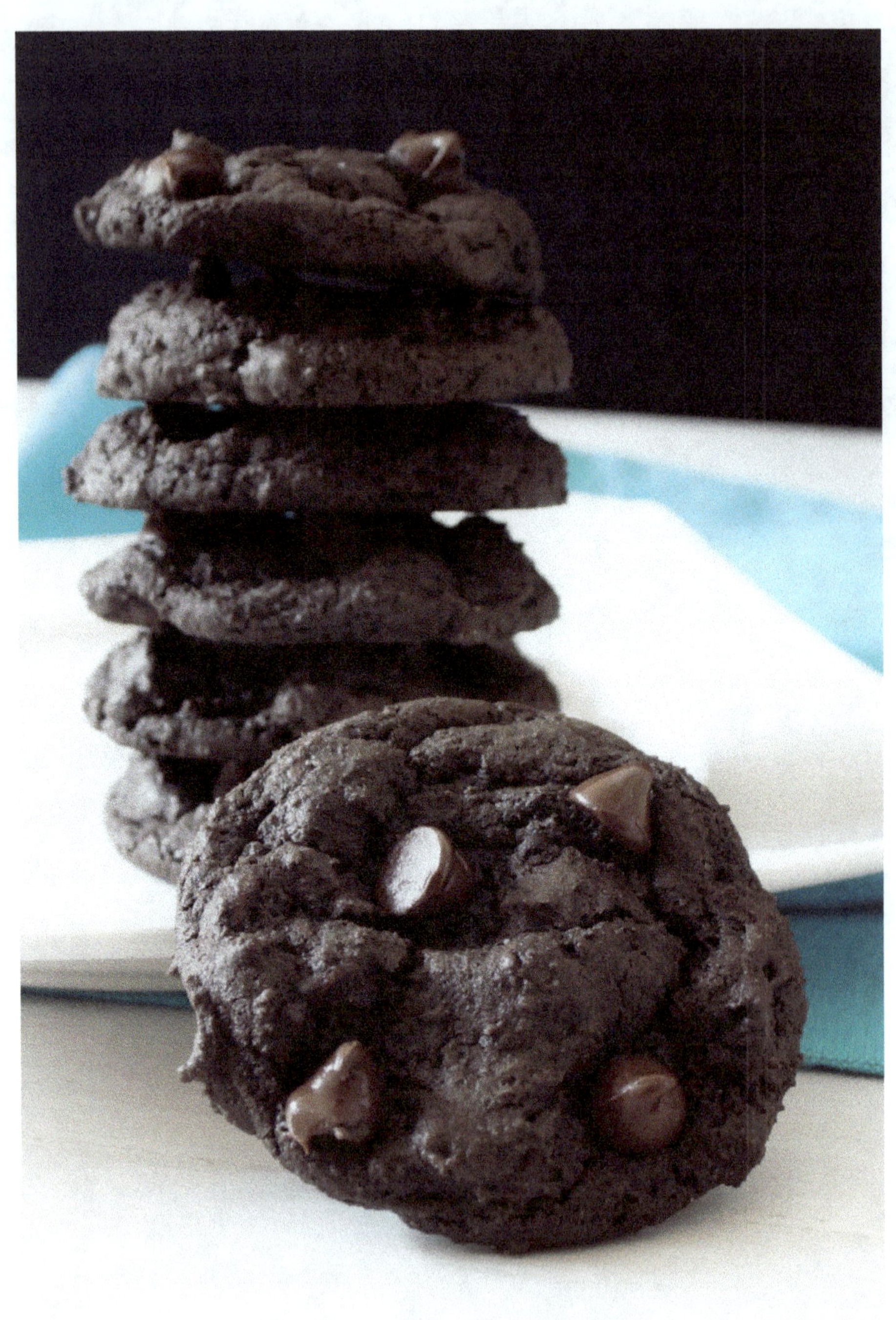

Chocolate Avocado Ice Cream

Servings: 6

Cooking Time: 0 Minutes

Ingredients:

- Large organic avocados, pitted: 2
- Erythritol, powdered: ½ cup
- Cocoa powder, organic and unsweetened: ½ cup
- Drops of liquid stevia: 25
- Vanilla extract, unsweetened: 2 teaspoons
- Coconut milk, full-fat and unsweetened: 1 cup
- Heavy whipping cream, full-fat: ½ cup
- Squares of chocolate, unsweetened and chopped: 6

Directions:

1. Scoop out the flesh from each avocado, place it in a bowl and add vanilla, milk, and cream and blend using an immersion blender until smooth and creamy.
2. Add remaining ingredients except for chocolate and mix until well combined and smooth.
3. Fold in chopped chocolate and let the mixture chill in the refrigerator for 8 to 12 hours or until cooled.
4. When ready to serve, let ice cream stand for 30 minutes at room temperature, then process it using an ice cream machine as per manufacturer instruction.
5. Serve immediately.

Nutrition Info: Calories: 216.7 Fat: 19.4 g Protein: 3.8 g Net Carbs: 3.7 g Fiber: 7.4 g

Marinated Strawberries

Servings: 6

Cooking Time: 35 Minutes

Ingredients:

- 4 cups (2 pints) strawberries
- 1 to 2 tbsps. sugar
- 2 tbsps. aged balsamic vinegar
- 2 tbsps. finely shredded fresh mint
- 1 tbsp. lemon juice
- 3 cups low-fat or fat-free vanilla frozen yogurt

Directions:

1. Cut off strawberry stems; cut strawberries in half or into quarters lengthwise if large. Mix together lemon juice, mint, balsamic vinegar, sugar, and strawberries in a medium bowl. Cover and let chill in the fridge for at least 20 minutes or up to 4 hours.

2. Over scoops of frozen yogurt, spoon the strawberry mixture to serve.

Nutrition Info: Calories: 166 calories; Total Carbohydrate: 33 g Cholesterol: 10 mg Total Fat: 2 g Protein: 5 g Sodium: 77 mg Saturated Fat: 1 g

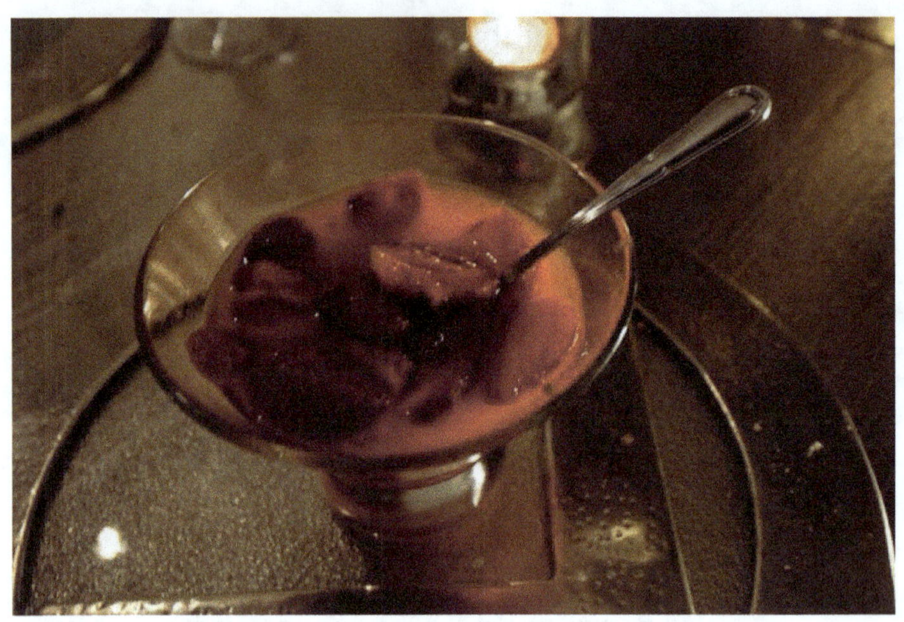

Tomato & Cheese In Lettuce Packets

Servings: 36

Cooking Time: 15 Minutes

Ingredients:

- ¼ pound Gruyere cheese, grated
- ¼ pound feta cheese, crumbled
- ½ tsp oregano
- 1 tomato, chopped
- ½ cup buttermilk
- ½ head lettuce

Directions:

1. In a bowl, mix feta and Gruyere cheese, oregano, tomato, and buttermilk.
2. Separate the lettuce leaves and put them on a serving platter. Divide the mixture between them, roll up, folding in the ends to secure and serve.

Nutrition Info: Calories 433 Fat: 32.5g Net Carbs: 6.6g Protein: 27.5g

Tofu & Chia Seed Pudding

Servings: 4

Cooking Time: 15 Minutes

Ingredients:

- 1-pound silken tofu, pressed and drained
- ¼ cup banana, peeled
- 3 tablespoons cacao powder
- 1 teaspoon vanilla extract
- 3 tablespoons chia seeds
- ¼ cup walnuts, chopped
- ¼ cup black raisins

Directions:

1. In a food processor, add tofu, banana, cocoa powder, and vanilla, and pulse till smooth and creamy.
2. Transfer into a large serving bowl and stir in chia seeds till well mixed.
3. Now, place the pudding in serving bowls evenly.

4. With plastic wraps, cover the bowls. Refrigerate to chill before serving.

5. Garnish with raspberries and serve.

Nutrition Info: Calories 188 Total Fat 10.4 g Saturated Fat 1.4 g Cholesterol 0 mg Sodium 42 mg Total Carbs 17.1 g Fiber 4.2 g Sugar 8.2 g Protein 12 g

Mango Mousse

Servings: 6

Cooking Time: 10 Minutes

Ingredients:

- 1 banana
- 2 mangoes, seeded, cubed, and peeled
- 2/3 cup plain yogurt
- 1 cup low-fat milk
- 1/8 cup unsweetened coconut
- What you will need from the store cupboard:
- 1 teaspoon vanilla extract
- 6 ice cubes
- 2 teaspoons honey

Directions:

1. Bring together the vanilla extract, yogurt, honey, ice cubes, mangoes and banana in your blender.
2. Blend until it becomes smooth.

3. Refrigerate for a couple of hours.

4. Pour into each dish before serving.

Nutrition Info: Calories 87, Carbohydrates 20g, Fiber 2g, Sugar 2g, Cholesterol 1mg, Total Fat 0g, Protein 2g

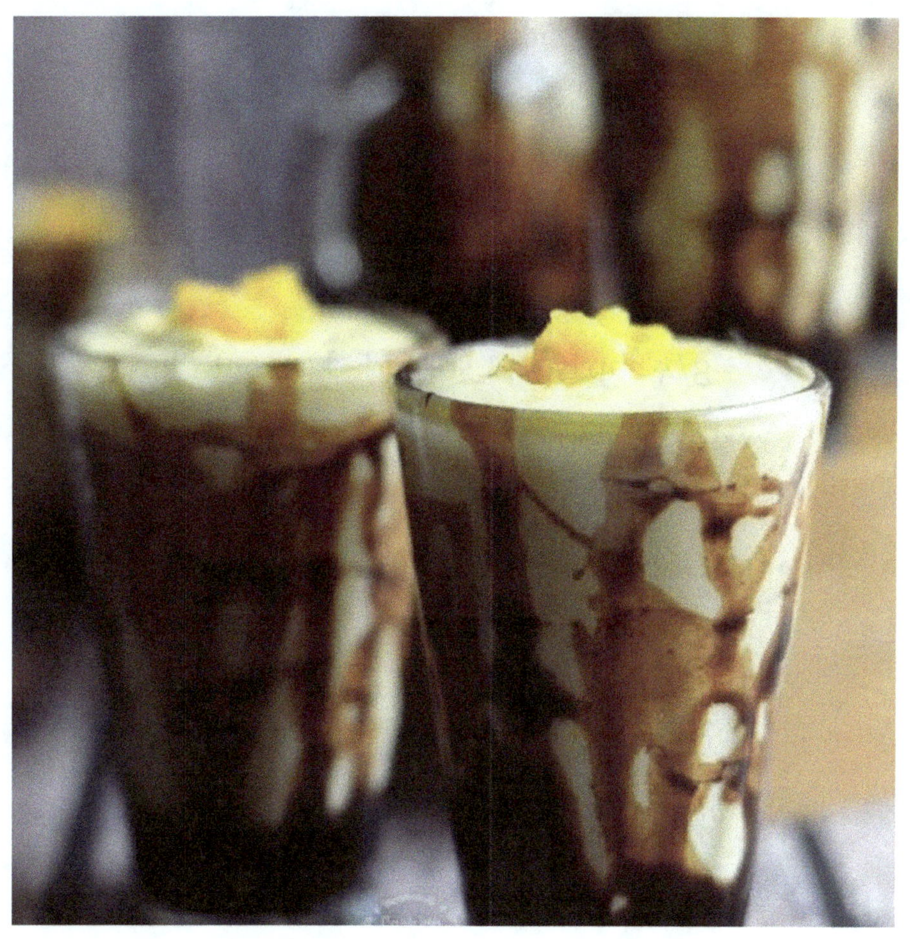

Nutty Wild Rice Salad

Servings: 8

Cooking Time: 40 Minutes

Ingredients:

- 2/3 cup uncooked wild rice
- cans (14 ounces) sauerkraut rinsed and well drained
- 1 medium apple peeled and chopped
- 3/4 cup celery chopped
- 3/4 cup carrot shredded (about 1 large carrot)
- 1/2 cup red onion finely chopped
- Dressing
- 1/2 cup sugar
- 1/3 cup cider vinegar
- 1 tbsp canola oil
- 1/4 tsp salt
- 1/4 tsp pepper
- 1 tbsp fresh parsley minced

- 1 tbsp fresh tarragon minced (or 1 tsp dried tarragon)
- 3/4 cup walnuts chopped, toasted

Directions:

1. Cook wild rice according to package directions. Cool completely.

2. In a large bowl, combine sauerkraut, apple, celery, carrot, onion and cooled rice. In a small bowl, whisk the first five dressing ingredients until sugar is dissolved; stir in herbs. Add to sauerkraut mixture; toss to combine.

3. Refrigerate, covered, at least 4 hours to allow flavours to blend. Stir in walnuts just before serving.

4. Tip: To toast nuts, bake in a shallow pan in a 350° oven for 5-10 minutes or cook in a skillet over low heat until lightly browned, stirring occasionally.

Nutrition Info: 300 calories 27.5g fat 6g protein 14.5g carbs 10g fiber 4.5g net carbs

Banana Split Sundae

Servings: 4

Cooking Time: 0 Minutes

Ingredients:

- 3 frozen, sliced overripe bananas (see Tip)
- 2 tbsps. peanut butter
- 1 tbsp. thawed frozen light whipped topping
- 1 tsp. sugar-free chocolate-flavor syrup
- 1 tsp. chopped peanuts
- 1 maraschino cherry

Directions:

1. Combine peanut butter and bananas in a food processor. Process with cover until almost no lumps remain. Scoop the mixture into sundae dishes.

2. Garnish top with whipped topping, maraschino cherry, peanuts and sugar-free chocolate-flavor syrup. Serve right away.

Nutrition Info: Calories: 166 calories Total Carbohydrate: 27 g Cholesterol: 0 mg Total Fat: 6 g Fiber: 3 g Protein: 3 g Sodium: 60 mg Sugar: 14 g Saturated Fat: 2 g

Tzatziki Dip With Cauliflower

Servings: 6

Cooking Time: 0 Minutes

Ingredients:

- ½ (8-ounce) package cream cheese, softened
- 1 cup sour cream
- 1 tablespoon ranch seasoning
- 1 English cucumber, diced
- 2 tablespoons chopped chives
- 2 cups cauliflower florets

Directions:

1. Beat the cream cheese with an electric mixer until creamy.
2. Add the sour cream and ranch seasoning, then beat until smooth.
3. Fold in the cucumbers and chives, then chill before serving with cauliflower florets for dipping.

Nutrition Info: 125 calories 10.5g fat 3g protein 5.5g carbs 1g fiber 4.5g net carbs

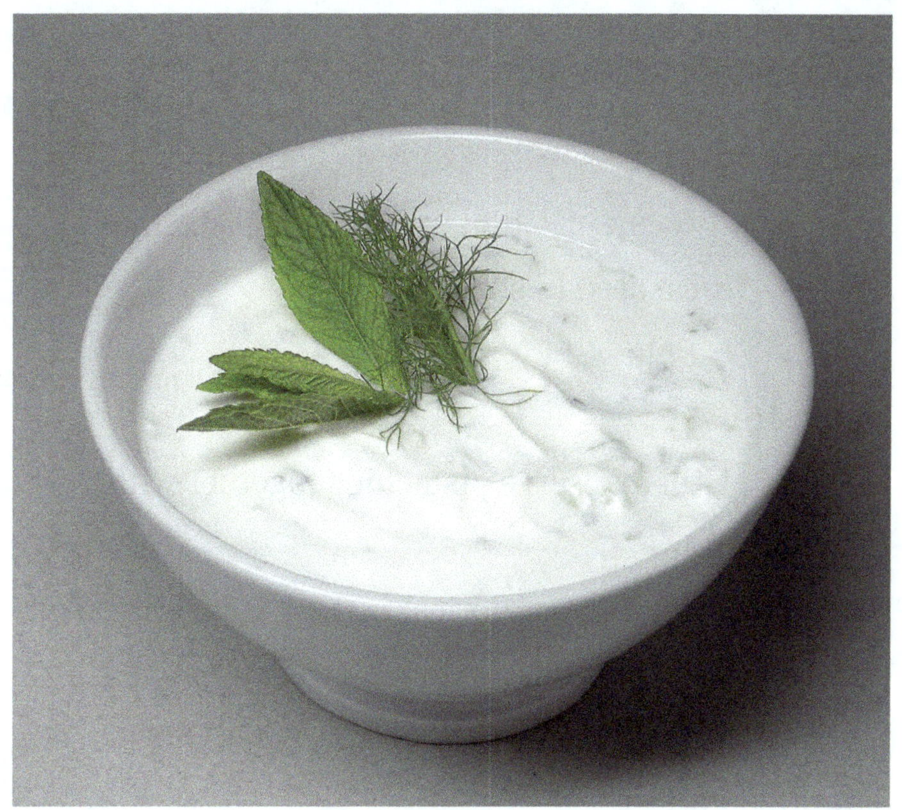

Plum & Pistachio Snack

Servings: 1

Cooking Time: 5 Minutes

Ingredients:

- ¼ cup unsalted dry-roasted pistachios (measured in shell)
- 1 plum

Directions:

1. Hull and serve pistachios together with plum.

Nutrition Info: Calories: 113 calories; Total Carbohydrate: 12 g Cholesterol: 0 mg Total Fat: 7 g Fiber: 2 g Protein: 4 g Sodium: 1 mg Sugar: 8 g Saturated Fat: 1 g

Fruity Tofu Smoothie

Servings: 2

Cooking Time: 10 Minutes

Ingredients:

- 12 ounces' silken tofu, pressed and drained
- 2 medium bananas, peeled
- 1½ cups fresh blueberries
- 1 tablespoon maple syrup
- 1½ cups unsweetened soymilk
- ¼ cup ice cubes

Directions:

1. Place all the ingredients in a high-speed blender and pulse until creamy.
2. Pour into two glasses and serve immediately.

Nutrition Info: Calories 398 Total Fat 8.6 g Saturated Fat 1.2 g Cholesterol 0 mg Sodium 58 mg Total Carbs 65 g Fiber 7 g Sugar 50.7 g Protein 19.9 g

Strawberry Mousse

Servings: 6

Ingredients:

- 1½ cups fresh strawberries, hulled
- 1 2/3 cups chilled unsweetened almond milk
- 2-3 drops liquid stevia
- 1 teaspoon organic vanilla extract

Directions:

1. In a food processor, add all the ingredients and pulse until smooth.
2. Transfer into serving bowls and serve.
3. Meal Prep Tip: Transfer the mousse into an airtight container. Cover the containers and refrigerate for up to 3 days.

Nutrition Info: Calories 25 Total Fat 1.1g Saturated Fat 0.1 g Cholesterol 0 mg Total Carbs 3.4 g Sugar 1.9 g Fiber 1 g Sodium 50 mg Potassium 109 mg Protein 0.5 g

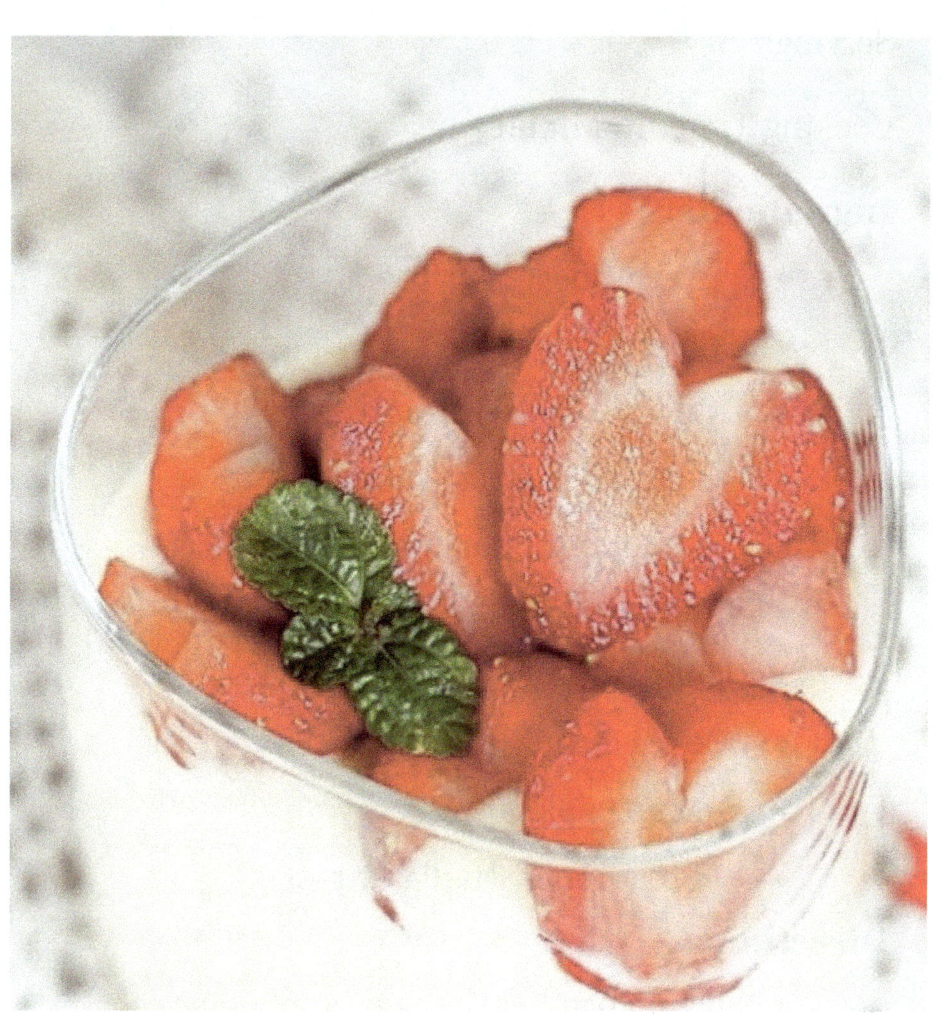

Raisin Apple Cake

Servings: 6

Cooking Time: 10 Minutes

Ingredients:

- 2 eggs, beaten
- ½ cup raisins
- ½ cup whole-wheat flour
- 1 cup all-purpose flour
- 1 teaspoon cinnamon, ground
- What you will need from the store cupboard:
- 2 teaspoons baking powder
- 1 cup applesauce
- 2 teaspoons vanilla extract

Directions:

1. Bring together the eggs, apple sauce, cinnamon, flour, baking powder, vanilla and raisins in your mixing bowl.
2. Use the batter to make small cakes.

3.   Now heat your girdle on medium heat.

4.   Fry the cakes. Make sure that both sides are brown.

Nutrition Info: Calories 203, Carbohydrates 41g, Fiber 3g, Sugar 1.4g, Cholesterol 62mg, Total Fat 1g, Protein 6g

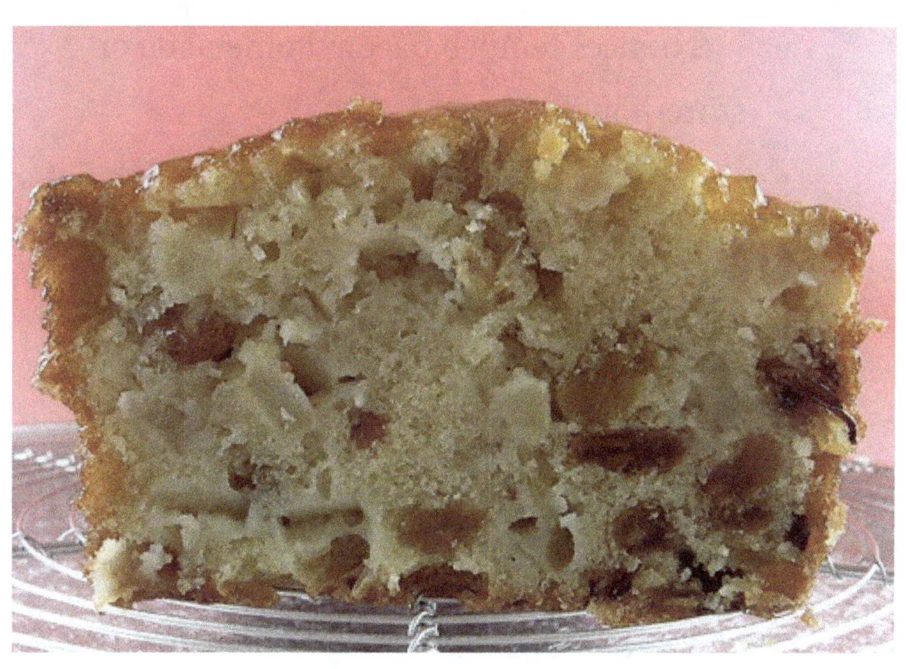

Avocado And Tempeh Bacon Wraps

Servings: 4

Cooking Time: 8 Minutes

Ingredients:

- 2 tablespoons extra-virgin olive oil
- 8 ounces tempeh bacon, homemade or store-bought
- 4 (10-inch) soft flour tortillas or lavish flat bread
- ¼cup vegan mayonnaise, homemade or store-bought
- 4 large lettuce leaves
- 2 ripe Hass avocados, pitted, peeled, and cut into ¼-inch slices
- 1 large ripe tomato, cut into ¼-inch slices

Directions:

1. Preparing the Ingredients
2. Cook the tempeh bacon until browned on both sides in a large skillet about 8 minutes. Remove from the heat and set aside.
3. Place 1 tortilla on a work surface. Spread with some of the mayonnaise and one-fourth of the lettuce and tomatoes.
4. Finish and Serve
5. Pit, peel, and thinly slice the avocado and place the slices on top of the tomato. Add the reserved tempeh bacon and roll up tightly. Repeat with remaining Ingredients and serve.

Nutrition Info: Fat: 24.3 g Protein: 11.7 g Carbohydrates: 16.7 g

Coco-macadamia Fat Bombs

Servings: 16

Cooking Time: 0 Minutes

Ingredients:

- 1 cup coconut oil
- 1 cup smooth almond butter
- ½ cup unsweetened cocoa powder
- ¼ cup coconut flour
- Liquid stevia extract, to taste
- 16 whole macadamia nuts, raw

Directions:

1. Melt the coconut oil and cashew butter together in a small saucepan.
2. Whisk in the cocoa powder, coconut flour, and liquid stevia to taste.
3. Remove from heat and let cool until it hardens slightly.
4. Divide the mixture into 16 even pieces.

5.   Roll each piece into a ball around a macadamia nut and chill until ready to eat.

Nutrition Info: 255 calories 25.5g fat 3.5g protein 7g carbs 3g fiber 4g net carbs

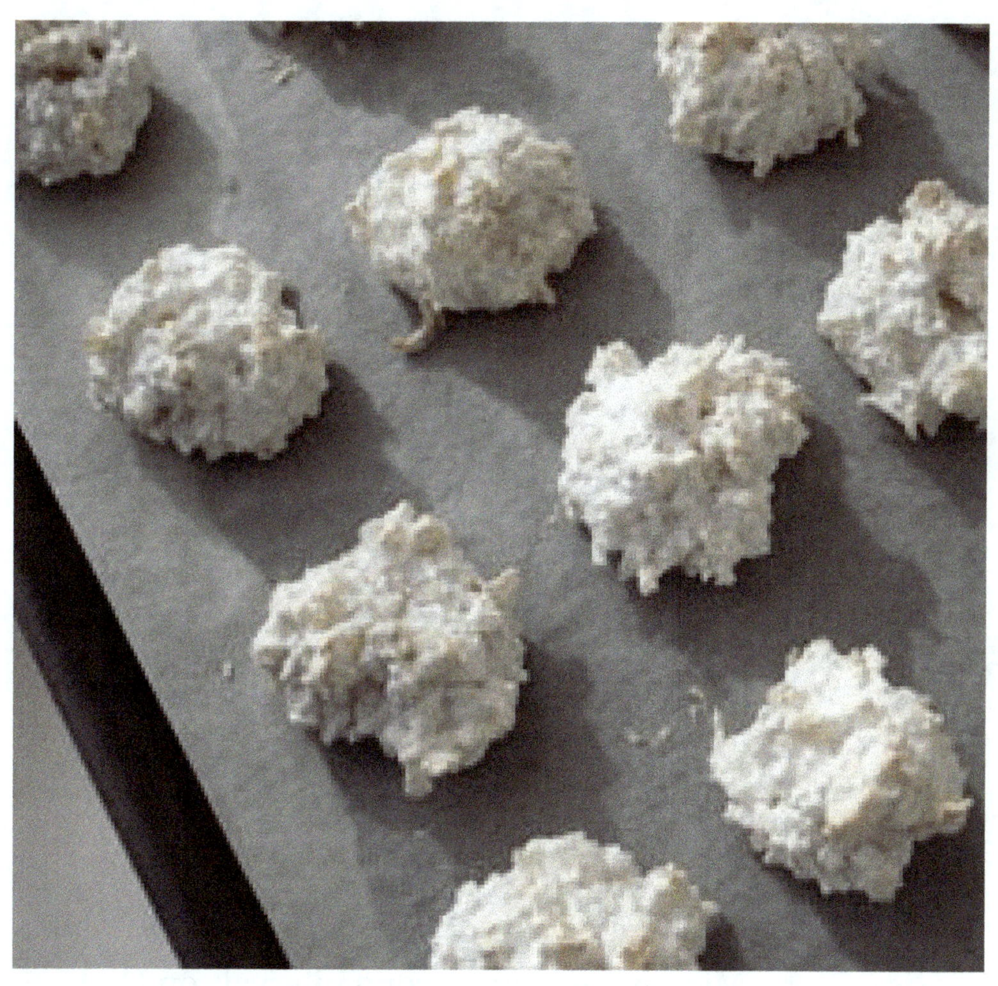

Chocolate-covered Prosecco Strawberries

Servings: 2

Cooking Time: 45 Minutes

Ingredients:

- 12 medium strawberries, rinsed and dried
- 2 cups prosecco or other sparkling wine
- ⅓ cup bittersweet chocolate chips (2 oz.)

Directions:

1. In a medium bowl, combine prosecco and strawberries. Keep the strawberries submerged by placing a bowl on top. Cover and place in the refrigerator overnight or for at least 8 hours.

2. Transfer the strawberries to a plate lined with paper towels and pat dry. In a microwave-safe bowl, put the chocolate chips. Microwave in 20-second intervals on High, stirring each interval, until chocolate is

melted, about 1 minute. Dip strawberries into
the chocolate and put them onto a plate lined
with waxed paper. Let sit in refrigerator until
the chocolate is firm, about 15 to 20 minutes.

Nutrition Info: Calories: 50 calories; Total
Carbohydrate: 7 g Cholesterol: 0 mg Total Fat: 3 g
Fiber: 1 g Protein: 1 g Sodium: 0 mg Sugar: 5 g
Saturated Fat: 1 g

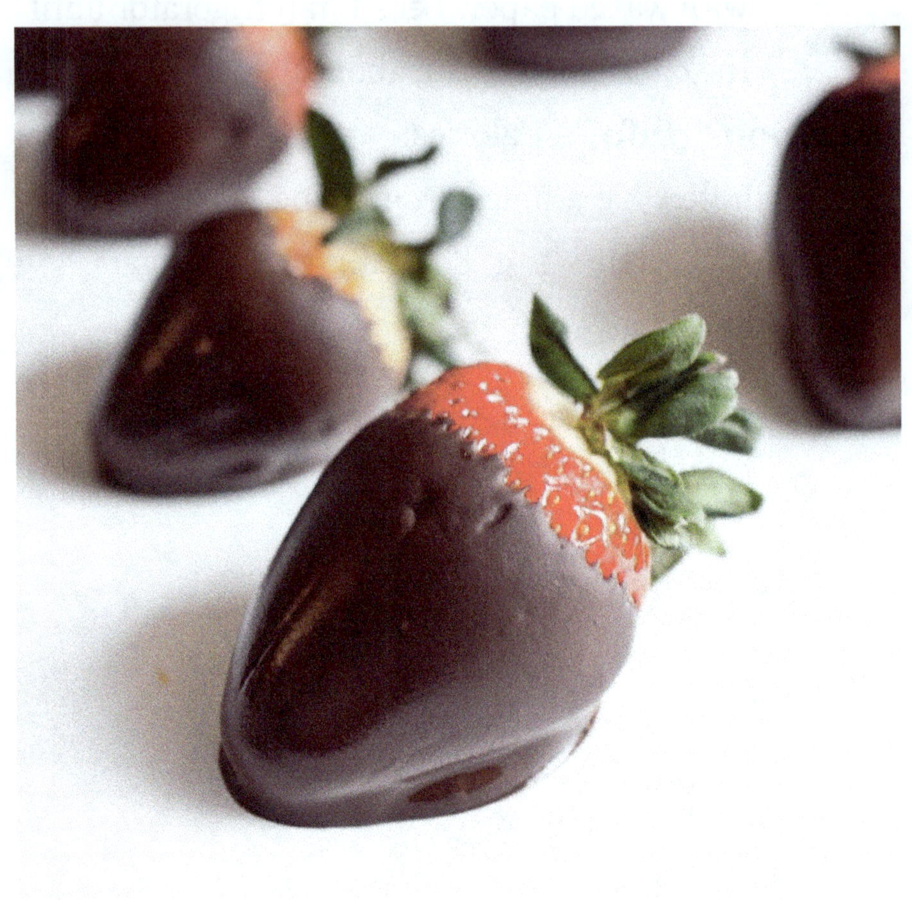

Pumpkin Spice Snack Balls

Servings: 10

Cooking Time: 10 Minutes

Ingredients:

- 1 ½ cups old-fashioned oats
- ½ cup chopped almonds
- ½ cup unsweetened shredded coconut
- ¾ cup canned pumpkin puree
- 2 tablespoons honey
- 2 teaspoons pumpkin pie spice
- ¼ teaspoon salt

Directions:

1. Preheat the oven to 300°F and line a baking sheet with parchment.
2. Combine the oats, almonds, and coconut on the baking sheet.
3. Bake for 8 to 10 minutes until browned, stirring halfway through.

4. Place the pumpkin, honey, pumpkin pie spice, and salt in a medium bowl.

5. Stir in the toasted oat mixture.

6. Shape the mixture into 20 balls by hand and place on a tray.

7. Chill until the balls are firm then serve.

Nutrition Info: Calories 170, Total Fat 9.8g, Saturated Fat 6g, Total Carbs 17.8g, Net Carbs 13.7g, Protein 3.8g, Sugar 5.2g, Fiber 4.1g, Sodium 64mg

Chocolatey Banana Shake

Servings: 2

Cooking Time: 10 Minutes

Ingredients:

- 2 medium frozen bananas, peeled
- 4 dates, pitted
- 4 tablespoons peanut butter
- 4 tablespoons rolled oats
- 2 tablespoons cacao powder
- 2 tablespoons chia seeds
- 2 cups unsweetened soymilk

Directions:

1. Place all the ingredients in a high-speed blender and pulse until creamy.
2. Pour into two glasses and serve immediately.

Nutrition Info: Calories 583 Total Fat 25.2 g Saturated Fat 4.8 g Cholesterol 0 mg Sodium 200 mg Total Carbs 75 g Fiber 15.3 g Sugar 37.8 g Protein 23.1 g

Chia Strawberry Pudding

Servings: 4

Cooking Time: 10 Minutes

Ingredients:

- 1 tsp unsweetened cocoa powder
- 5 tbsp chia seeds
- 2 tbsp xylitol
- 1 1/2 tsp vanilla
- 1 ½ cups strawberries, chopped
- 1 cup unsweetened coconut milk
- Pinch of salt

Directions:

1. In a saucepan, combine together strawberries, ½ cup water, xylitol, vanilla, and salt and simmer over medium heat for 5-10 minutes.
2. Mash strawberries with a fork.
3. Add coconut milk and stir to combine.

4. Add chia seeds and mix well and let it sit for
    5 minutes.

5. Pour pudding mixture in serving glasses.

6. Sprinkle cocoa powder on top of chia
    pudding.

7. Place in refrigerator for 1 hour.

8. Serve chilled and enjoy.

Nutrition Info: Calories 211 Fat 17.4 g Carbohydrates
11 g Sugar 4.9 g Protein 3.8 g Cholesterol 0 mg

Chocolate Banana Cake

Servings: 12

Cooking Time: 20 Minutes

Ingredients:

- 2 eggs
- 1 cup ripe bananas, mashed
- 1-1/3 cups all-purpose flour
- 3 tablespoons cocoa, crushed
- 1 cup low-fat milk
- What you will need from the store cupboard:
- 2 teaspoons vanilla extract
- ½ teaspoon baking soda
- 1 teaspoon baking powder
- 1/3 cup butter
- ½ teaspoon salt
- ½ cup of water
- Cooking spray

Directions:

1. Preheat your oven to 350 °F. Apply cooking spray to your baking pan.
2. Add butter until it is fluffy and light.
3. Add the eggs and vanilla (1 at a time). Beat after each addition.
4. Now stir the water in.
5. Whisk together the milk, flour, baking powder, cocoa, salt, and baking soda.
6. Add this to the creamed mix. Combine well.
7. Stir the bananas in.
8. Place in your pan and bake.

Nutrition Info: Calories 169, Carbohydrates 25g, Fiber 1g, Sugar 1g, Cholesterol 45mg, Total Fat 6g, Protein 4g

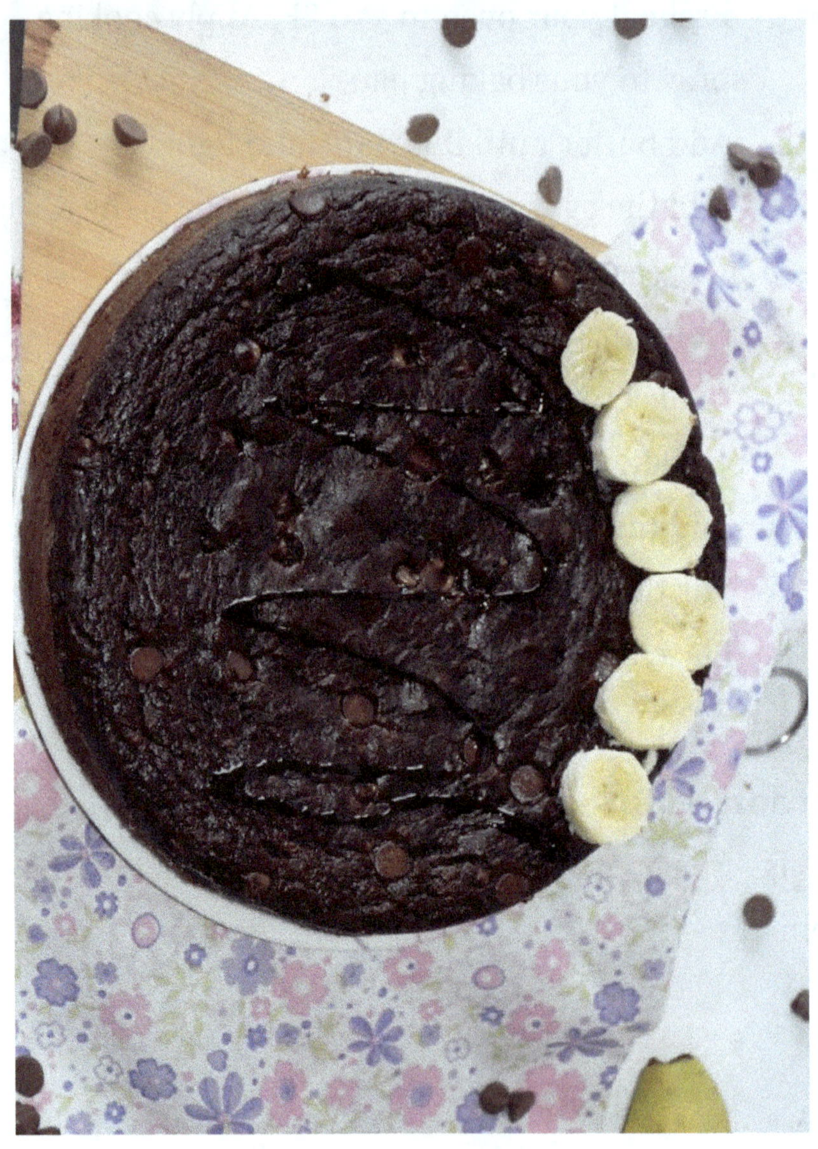

Delicious Egg Cups With Cheese & Spinach

Servings: 2

Cooking Time: 10 Minutes

Ingredients:

- 4 eggs
- 1 tbsp fresh parsley, chopped
- ¼ cup cheddar cheese, shredded
- ¼ cup spinach, chopped
- Salt and black pepper to taste

Directions:

1. Grease muffin cups with cooking spray. In a bowl, whisk the eggs and add in the rest of the ingredients. Season with salt and black pepper. Fill ¾ parts of each muffin cup with the egg mixture.

2. Bake in the oven for 15 minutes at 390 F. Serve warm!

Nutrition Info: Calories: 232 Fat 14.3g Net Carbs 1.5g Protein 16.2g

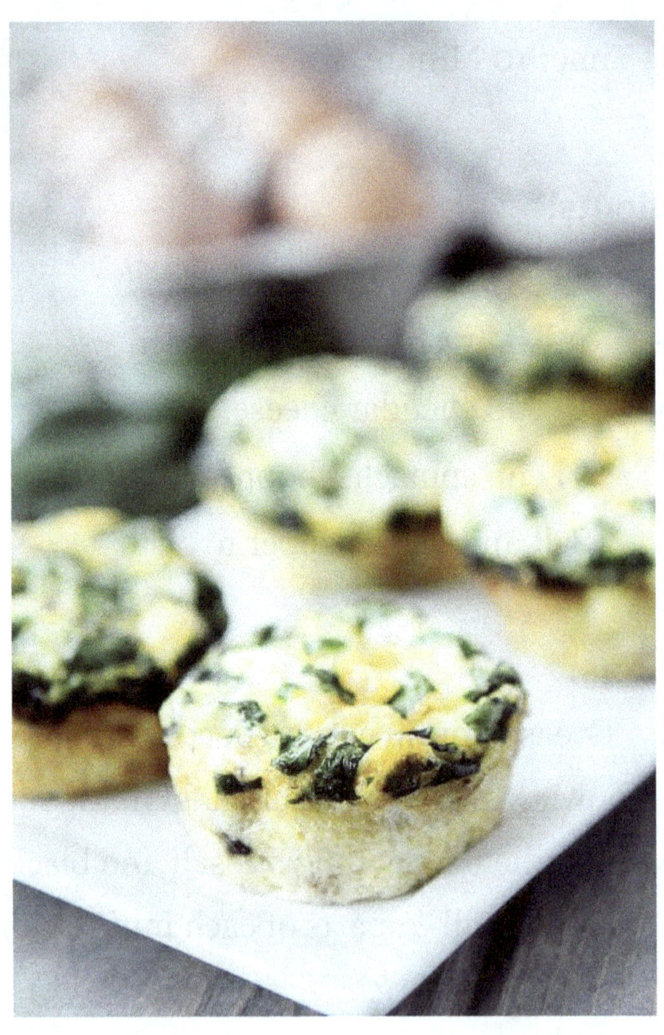

Lemon Custard

Servings: 4

Cooking Time: 3 Hours

Ingredients:

- 2 cups whipping cream or coconut cream
- 5 egg yolks
- 1 tablespoon lemon zest
- 1 teaspoon vanilla extract
- 1/4 cup fresh lemon juice, squeezed
- 1/2 teaspoon liquid stevia
- Lightly sweetened whipped cream

Directions:

1. Whisk egg yolks together with lemon zest, liquid stevia, lemon zest and vanilla in a bowl, and then whisk in heavy cream.
2. Divide the mixture among 4 small jars or ramekins.

3. To the bottom of a slow cooker add a rack, and then add ramekins on top of the rack and add enough water to cover half of ramekins.

4. Close the lid and cook for 3 hours on low. Remove ramekins.

5. Let cool to room temperature, and then place into the refrigerator to cool completely for about 3 hours.

6. When through, top with the whipped cream and serve. Enjoy!

Nutrition Info: 319 calories; 30 g fat; 3 g total carbs; 7 g protein

Yogurt Cheesecake

Servings: 8

Cooking Time: 35 Minutes

Ingredients:

- 2½ cups fat-free plain Greek yogurt
- 6-8 drops liquid stevia
- 3 egg whites
- 1/3 cup cacao powder
- ¼ cup arrowroot starch
- 1 teaspoon organic vanilla extract
- Pinch of sea salt

Directions:

1. Preheat the oven to 35 degrees F. Grease a 9-inch cake pan.
2. In a large bowl, add all ingredients and mix until well combined.
3. Place the mixture into the prepared pan evenly.
4. Bake for about 30-35 minutes.

5. Remove from oven and let it cool completely.

6. Refrigerate to chill for about 3-4 hours or until set completely.

7. Cut into 8 equal sized slices and serve.

8. Meal Prep Tip: With foil pieces, wrap the cheesecake slices and refrigerate for about 1-3 days. Reheat in the microwave before serving.

Nutrition Info: Calories 74 Total Fat 0.9g Saturated Fat 0.4 g Cholesterol 2 mg Total Carbs 8.5 g Sugar 3 g Fiber 1.1 g Sodium 89 mg Potassium 21 mg Protein 9.5 g

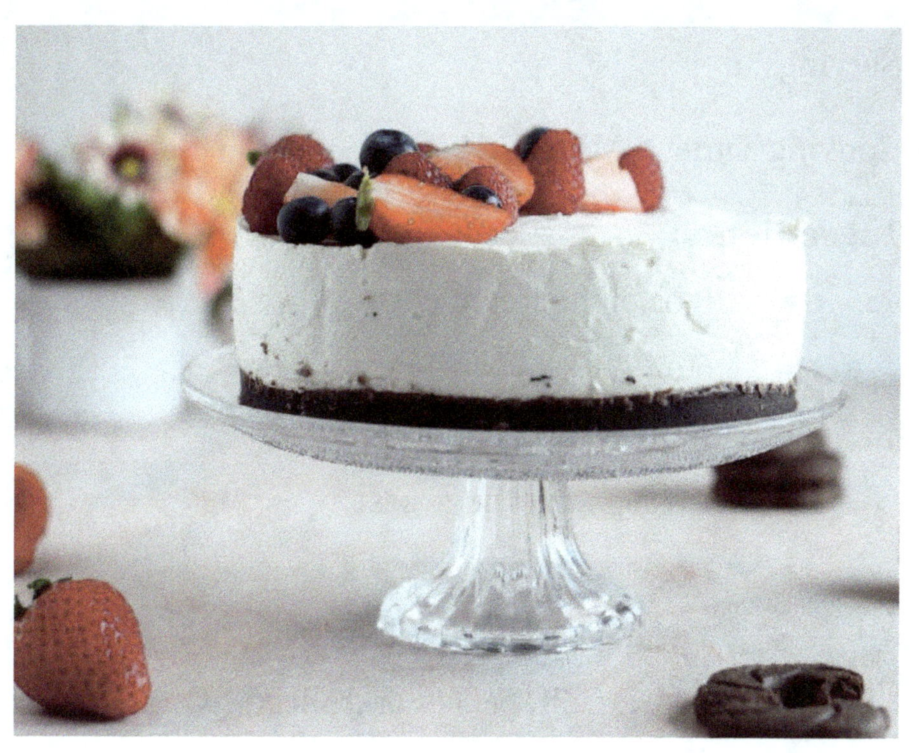

Fruit Salad

Servings: 6

Cooking Time: 0 Minute

Ingredients:

- 8 oz. light cream cheese
- 6 oz. Greek yogurt
- 1 tablespoon honey
- 1 teaspoon orange zest
- 1 teaspoon lemon zest
- 1 orange, sliced into sections
- 3 kiwi fruit, peeled and sliced
- 1 mango, cubed
- 1 cup blueberries

Directions:

1. Beat cream cheese using an electric mixer.
2. Add yogurt and honey.
3. Beat until smooth.
4. Stir in the orange and lemon zest.
5. Toss the fruits to mix.

6.   Divide in glass jars.

7.   Top with the cream cheese mixture.

Nutrition Info: Calories 131 Total Fat 3 g Saturated Fat 2 g Cholesterol 9 mg Sodium 102 mg Total Carbohydrate 23 g Dietary Fiber 3 g Total Sugars 18 g Protein 5 g Potassium 234 mg

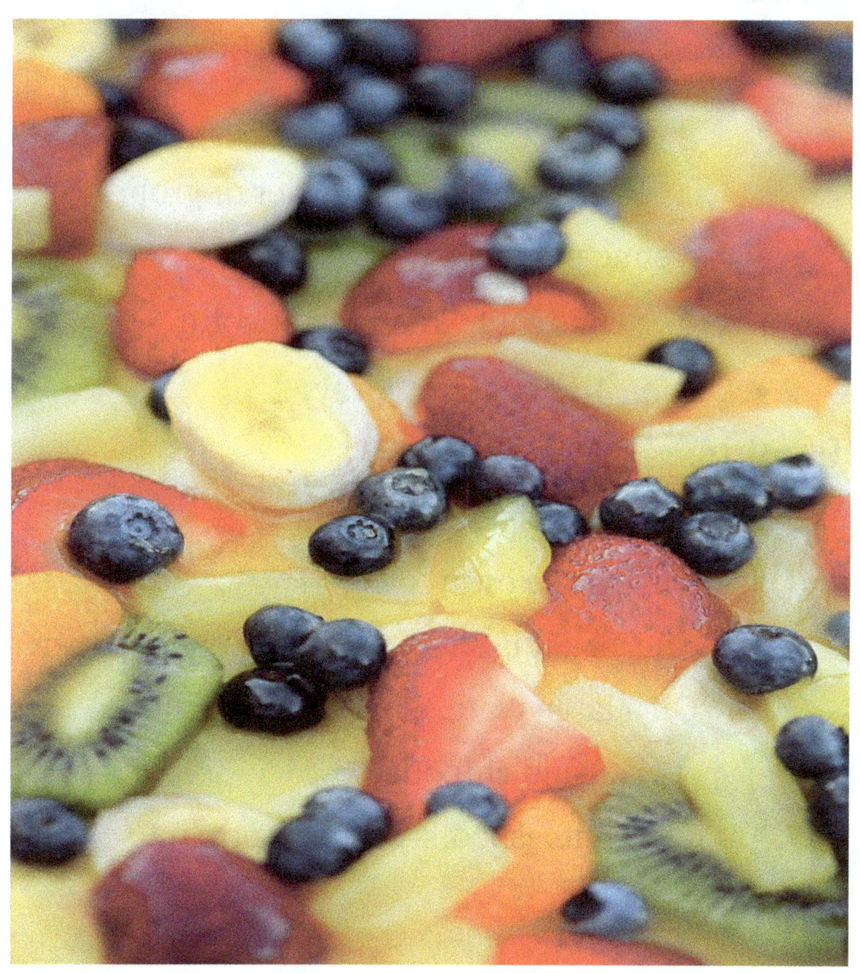

Risotto Bites

Servings: 12

Cooking Time: 20 Minutes

Ingredients:

- ½ cup panko bread crumbs
- 1 teaspoon paprika
- 1 teaspoon chipotle powder or ground cayenne pepper
- 1½ cups cold Green Pea Risotto
- Nonstick cooking spray

Directions:

1. Preparing the Ingredients
2. Preheat the oven to 425°F.
3. Line a baking sheet with parchment paper.
4. On a large plate, combine the panko, paprika, and chipotle powder. Set aside.
5. Roll 2 tablespoons of the risotto into a ball.

6.   Gently roll in the bread crumbs, and place on
     the prepared baking sheet. Repeat to make a
     total of 12 balls.

7.   Bake

8.   Spritz the tops of the risotto bites with
     nonstick cooking spray and bake for 15-20
     minutes until they begin to brown.

9.   Finish and Serve

10. Cool completely before storing in a large
     airtight container in a single layer (add a
     piece of parchment paper for a second layer),
     or in a plastic freezer bag.

Nutrition Info: Calories: 100 Fat: 2g Protein: 6g
Carbohydrates: 17g Fiber: 5g Sugar: 2g Sodium: 165mg

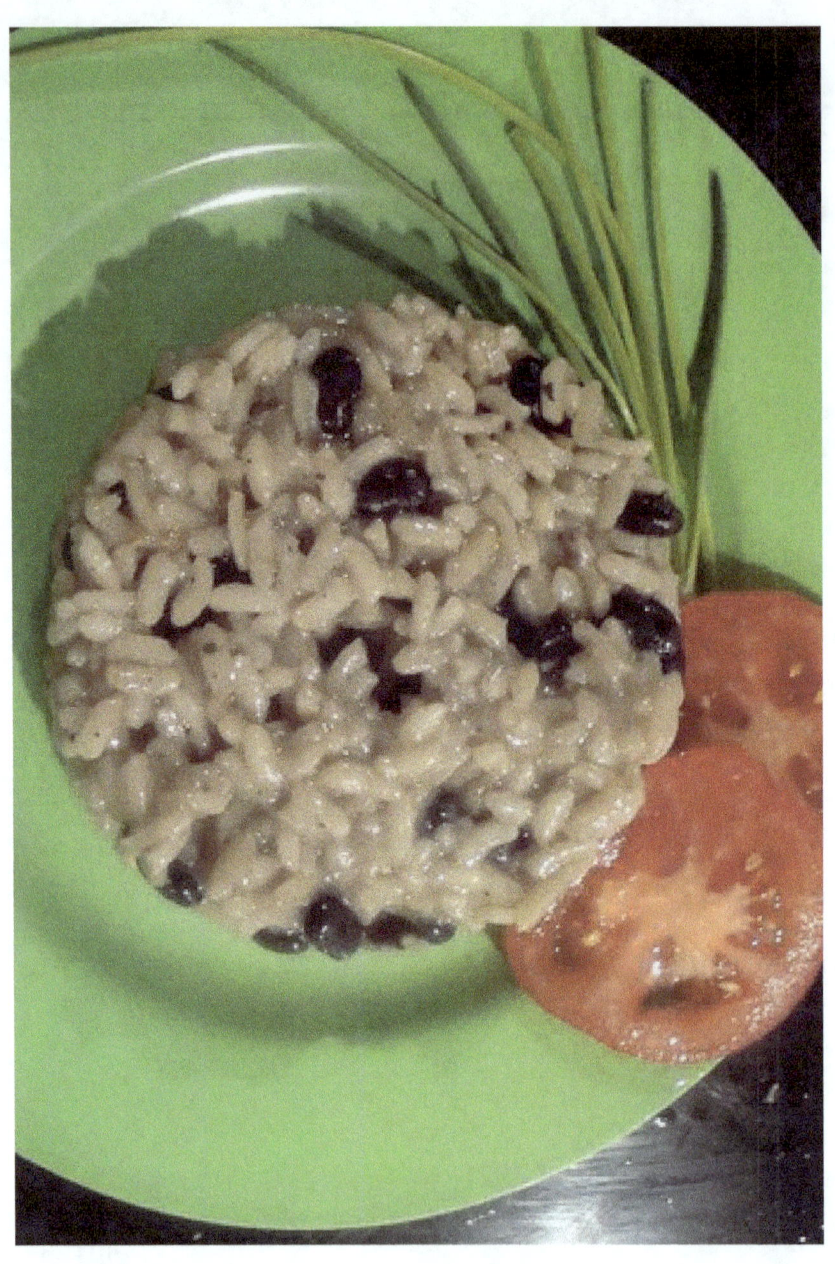

Grilled Avocado Hummus Paninis

Servings: 4

Cooking Time: 10 Minutes

Ingredients:

- 4 whole-wheat sandwich thins, split in half
- 1/3 cup roasted red pepper hummus
- ½ medium avocado, pitted and sliced thin
- Fresh ground pepper
- 1 cup fresh baby spinach, chopped
- 2 ounces feta cheese

Directions:

1. Lay the sandwich thins out flat.
2. Spread the hummus evenly on both sides of each sandwich thin.
3. Layer the avocado slices on the bottom of each sandwich thin and season with fresh ground black pepper.
4. Top each sandwich with ¼ cup spinach and ½ ounce cheese.

5. Add the top to each sandwich and press down lightly.

6. Grease a large skillet with cooking spray and heat over medium heat.

7. Add one or two sandwiches and place a heavy skillet on top.

8. Cook for 2 minutes or until the bottoms are toasted.

9. Flip the sandwiches and repeat on the other side. Cut in half to serve.

Nutrition Info: Calories 230, Total Fat 11.2g, Saturated Fat 3.2g, Total Carbs 27.8g, Net Carbs 19.2g, Protein 8.5g, Sugar 3.5g, Fiber 8.6g, Sodium 508mg

Cauliflower Muffin

Servings: 4

Cooking Time: 30 Minutes

Ingredients:

- 2,5 cup cauliflower
- 2/3 cup ham
- 2,5 cups of cheese
- 2/3 cup champignon
- 1,5 tbsp. flaxseed
- 3 eggs
- 1/4 tsp. salt
- 1/8 tsp. pepper

Directions:

1. Preheat oven to 375 F.
2. Put muffin liners in a 12-muffin tin.
3. Combine diced cauliflower, ground flaxseed, beaten eggs, cup diced ham, grated cheese, and diced mushrooms, salt, pepper.
4. Divide mixture rightly between muffin liners.

5. Bake 30 Minutes.

6. This is a great lunch for the whole family.

Nutrition Info: Calories 116 / Protein 10 g / Fat 7 g / Carbs 3 g

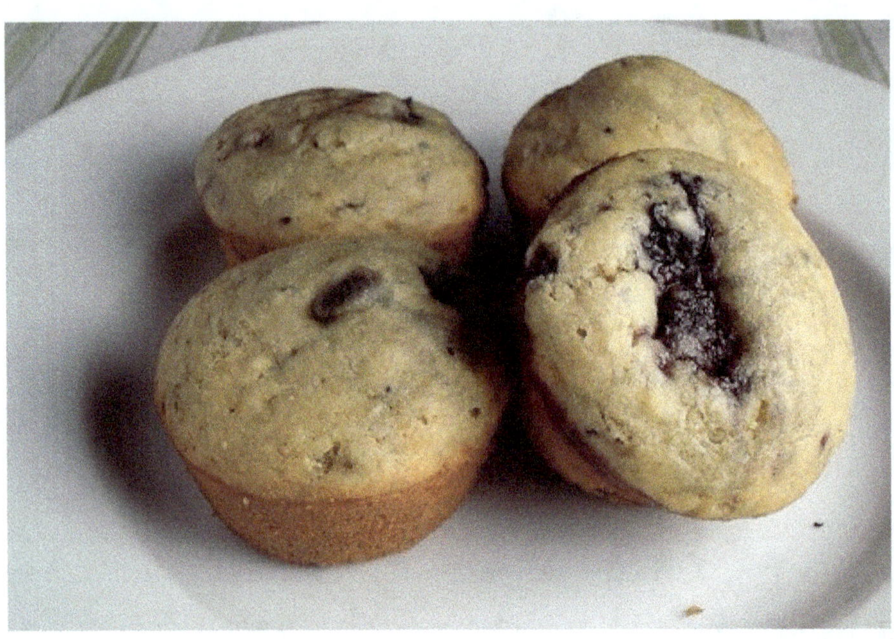

Bok Choy Soup

Servings: 4

Cooking Time: 25 Minutes

Ingredients:

- 2 tablespoons coconut oil, melted
- 1-pound bok choy, torn
- 2 shallots, chopped
- 4 cups chicken stock
- 1 cup heavy cream
- 1 tablespoon cilantro, chopped
- A pinch of salt and black pepper
- ½ teaspoon nutmeg, ground

Directions:

1. Heat up a pot with the oil over medium heat, add the shallots and sauté for 5 minutes.
2. Add the bok choy and the other ingredients, bring to a simmer and cook over medium heat for 20 minutes.

3.   Blend the soup using an immersion blender, divide into bowls and serve.

Nutrition Info: calories 194 fat 18.4 fiber 1.4 carbs 5.4 protein 3.2

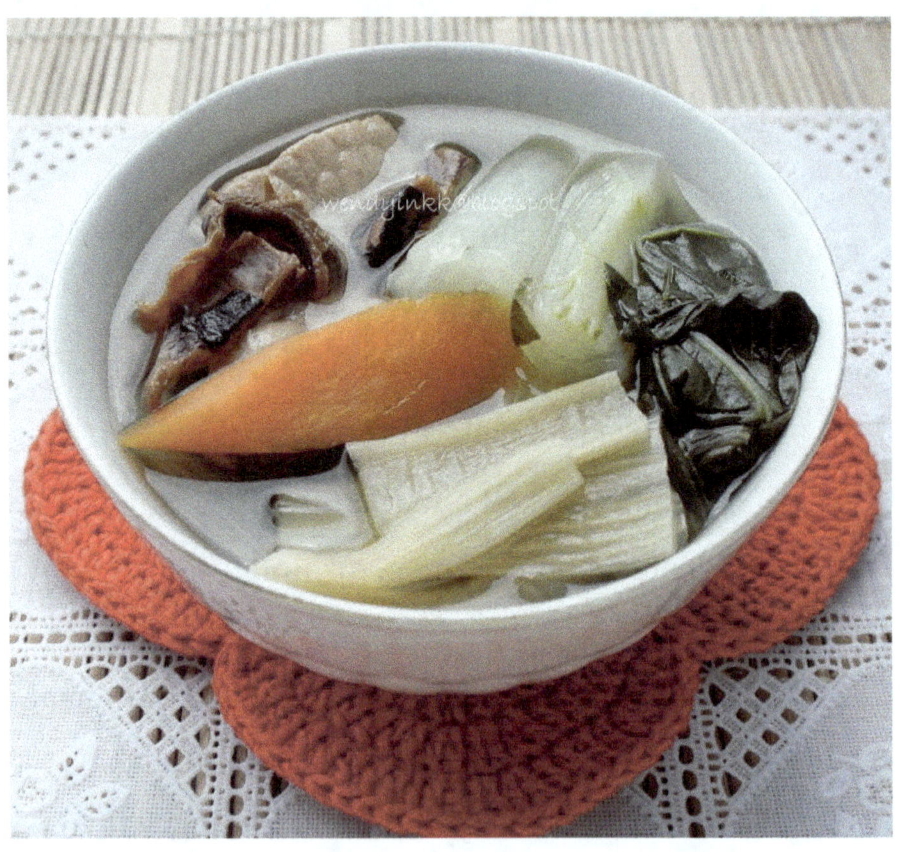

Stuffed Mushrooms

Servings: 4

Cooking Time: 20 Minutes

Ingredients:

- 4 Portobello Mushrooms, large
- 1/2 cup Mozzarella Cheese, shredded
- 1/2 cup Marinara, low-sugar
- Olive Oil Spray

Directions:

1. Preheat the oven to 375 F.
2. Take out the dark gills from the mushrooms with the help of a spoon.
3. Keep the mushroom stem upside down and spoon it with two tablespoons of marinara sauce and mozzarella cheese.
4. Bake for 18 minutes or until the cheese is bubbly.

Nutrition Info: Calories – 113kL; Fat – 6g; Carbohydrates – 4g; Protein – 7g; Sodium – 14mg

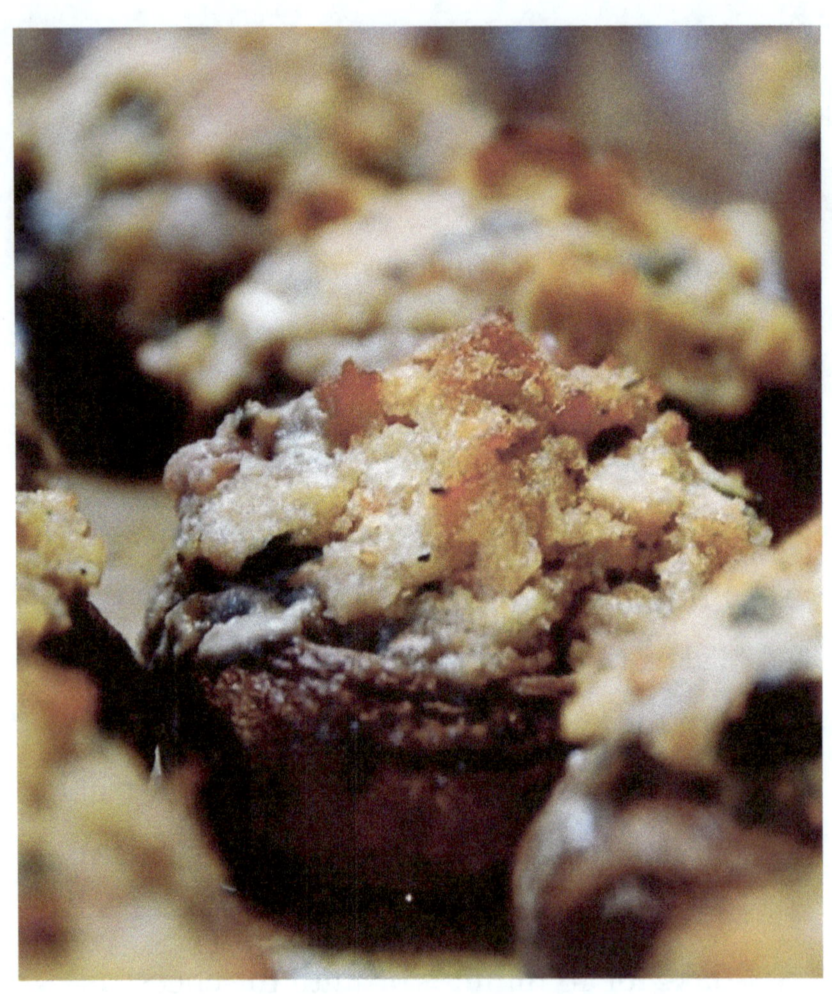

Roasted Salmon With Lemon

Servings: 6

Cooking Time: 25 Minutes

Ingredients:

- 1 salmon whole-side fillet, skin on
- 2 T. lemon juice
- 1 bunch fresh dill, chopped
- 4 T. butter
- 2 T. white wine
- 1/2 tsp. kosher salt
- 1/4 tsp. freshly ground black pepper

Directions:

1. Allow salmon to come to room temperature before baking. Preheat oven to 425°F. Mix dill and lemon juice in a small bowl. Lay fillet skin-side down on a parchment-lined baking sheet and cover with lemon-dill mixture. Top with butter, white wine, salt, and pepper.

Bake uncovered until the fish flakes easily with a fork, about 20-25 minutes.

Nutrition Info: Calories: 146.7 Fat: 10.9g Cholesterol: 49.1mg Sodium: 237.3mg Potassium: 269.5mg Carbohydrates: 0.8g Dietary Fiber: 0.1g Sugars: 0.2g Protein: 10.3g

White Spinach Pizza With Cauliflower Crust

Servings: 1 10-inch Pizza

Cooking Time: 25 Minutes

Ingredients:

- 1 head cauliflower, trimmed and chopped
- 2 eggs, beaten
- 2 c. shredded mozzarella cheese, divided
- 1/4 c. grated Parmesan cheese
- 2 tsp. Italian seasoning
- 3 T. extra virgin olive oil
- 1/2 c. shredded provolone cheese
- 3/4 c. whole milk ricotta cheese
- 3 cloves garlic, minced
- 1/4 c. thinly sliced red onion
- 1 c. baby spinach, washed

Directions:

1. To make the crust, pulse cauliflower florets in a food processor until they resemble rice. Microwave, covered loosely, for 5 minutes. Drain cauliflower in paper towel or cheesecloth, wringing out the towel to remove as much moisture as possible. Mix drained cauliflower with eggs, 1/2 cup of the mozzarella, Parmesan, and Italian seasoning. Press into a 10-inch round (or 10x15-inch rectangle) and bake at 425°F for 10-15 minutes. Brush crust with olive oil and top with remaining mozzarella, provolone, ricotta, garlic, red onion, and spinach. Bake for an additional 10 minutes or until the cheese is melted. This crust recipe will work with any toppings.

Nutrition Info: Calories: 350.3 Fat: 25.6g Cholesterol: 116.7mg Sodium: 558.7mg Potassium: 415.8mg Carbohydrates: 9.3g Dietary Fiber: 2.8g Sugars: 0.8g Protein: 22.4g

Chickpea, Tuna, And Kale Salad

Servings: 1

Cooking Time: None

Ingredients:

- 2 ounces fresh kale
- 2 tablespoons fat-free honey mustard dressing
- 1 (3-ounce) pouch tuna in water, drained
- 1 medium carrot, shredded
- Salt and pepper

Directions:

1. Trim the thick stems from the kale and cut into bite-sized pieces.
2. Toss the kale with the dressing in a salad bowl.
3. Top with tuna, chickpeas, and carrots. Season with salt and pepper to serve.

Nutrition Info: Calories 215, Total Fat 0.6g, Saturated Fat 0g, Total Carbs 28.1g, Net Carbs 23.6g, Protein 22.5g, Sugar 16g, Fiber 4.5g, Sodium 1176mg

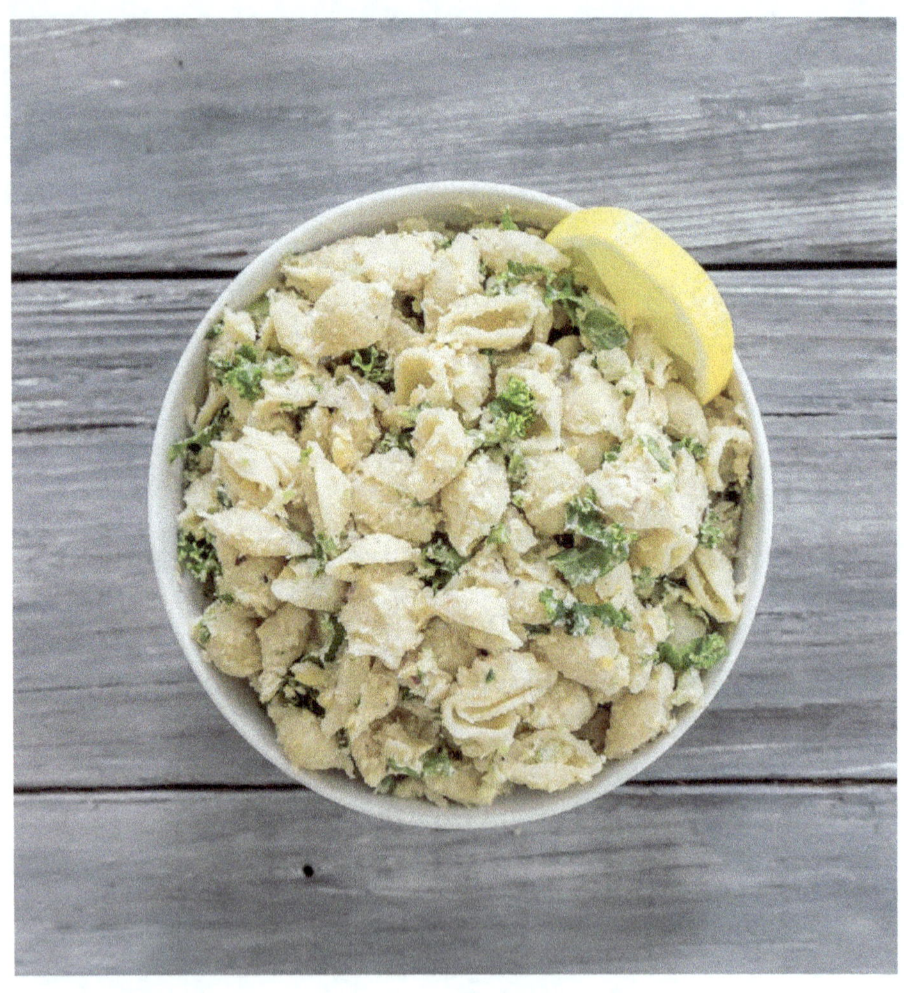

www.ingramcontent.com/pod-product-compliance
Lightning Source LLC
Chambersburg PA
CBHW071446030726

47593CB00003B/920